THE TRAP

SEX, SOCIAL MEDIA, AND SURVEILLANCE CAPITALISM

JEWELS JADE

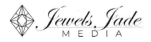

Jewels Jade
M E D I A

To my family.

You can't go back and change the beginning, but you can start where you are and change the ending.

— C.S. Lewis

PART I

1

LET US "PREY"

Though I have plenty of reasons for wanting to write this book, probably the largest one is this: who better than someone like me to tell the story?

I have worked in virtually every area of the adult entertainment industry for the past twenty years. I know how it operates, and, more importantly, how drastically it has changed...and not for the better.

Most of the people who work in adult entertainment don't last long, certainly not for as many years as I have. Sadly, sex workers have a notoriously short life span. Either they age out, burn out, or give out. Tragically, this means there are only a handful of us even left to be the truth-sayers. The problem is that most survivors are too shattered, too scared, and too dependent on a predatory system. We are frequently too ashamed to dare break ranks to offer an insider's view into the vast and ever-shifting labyrinth that is the porn industry.

Times are changing, though, and I hope you will find this book different from anything you have ever read, especially about business, technology, culture, and pornography.

This book actually is not about porn. It isn't about adult entertainment or the sex trade either, at least not as we traditionally know them. What if I told you that over the past two decades, a digital imposter I call the *Trap* has been steadily dismantling, absorbing, and replacing the adult industry right under our noses?

This process has been so subtle that most people, me included, didn't grasp the full impact of this metamorphosis until the Trap had already grown into one of the wealthiest, most powerful and influential forces on the planet. Though we will discuss this in far deeper detail later in the book, for now, all you need to know is that the Trap will still claim it's the same old porn industry we have always known **because it literally cannot afford for people to see the truth.**

The Trap wants people taking sides, labeling, and fighting because that is how it escapes scrutiny. I'm not saying pro-porn or anti-porn people don't both have valid points of view. Rather, I'm saying we have a much, much bigger problem that has completely evaded our notice.

The Trap twists *sexual freedom* and *empowerment* into serving as camouflage. It uses pop culture and pop psychology to convince us it is harmless and natural, not a dangerous mutation. It takes shameless advantage of human weaknesses and our desire to be a more sex-positive culture. All one needs to do is a quick scan of modern women's magazines, blogs, and articles to see the Trap's influence.

Want to improve your relationship? Spice up your marriage? Enjoy better sex? Hop online! Scroll some adult sites, watch some porn together, and embrace some fetish fun to add in that erotic zest. Even porn sites paint their own idyllic fiction for the public. Pornhub, one of the largest online porn sites, goes so far as to tout their own expert to emphasize how what they offer is positive and beneficial. From Pornhub's 2019 Year in Review[1]:

According to Dr. Laurie Betito of the Sexual Wellness Center:

It seems that people are looking for more realistic depictions of sex. 'Real' people vs. actors seems to be the draw. It's interesting that more and more people are putting themselves out there as amateurs. Sex has become so much less taboo that those who get a kick out of exhibitionism can do so with very little experience or equipment. The message is: anyone can be a porn star![2]

Perhaps Dr. Betito makes some reasonable observations, yet her message conveniently fails to mention any possible downsides. Why would she? She is there as a marketing tactic to legitimize the stance that Pornhub isn't simply there to make a profit. Rather, it's also performing a public service. I find this one-sided opinion to be fairly common with those who promote porn.

What is missing, though? Where are the warnings of potential side-effects and consequences not only for performers, but also for the audience?

There aren't any.

Disturbingly, in modern times, positive sexuality and a thrilling sex life alone are posited as somehow inadequate. Reading between the lines, the porn industry's mission statement surreptitiously skates across the thin barrier separating bedroom intimacy and public performance. The message, at least from sites like Pornhub, joining their roster of entertainers—even if on the amateur level—is where the real fun resides. For the truly liberated, exhibitionism and sexual play are good, safe, and healthy for all to enjoy. Everyone is happy and no harm done.

Sure.

While I know of performers who have chosen to be adult entertainers because they enjoy sex work as well as the myriad of benefits —high pay, flexible schedule, travel, financial independence, and early retirement to name a few—these are professionals who understand the business of the sex business. They have come to accept the good and the bad and operate on their own terms. They harness the advantages and parlay those into a better future, such as a robust investment portfolio, real estate holdings, higher education, or even opening their own establishments. These performers, however, are a very slim minority in twenty-first century porn. As you will see, the black hole of the internet is steadily devouring this segment of stars as well as gobbling up any bonuses these unique entertainers have historically enjoyed.

I believe that taking sides as pro-porn, anti-porn, or even middle-of-the-road-sometimes-porn is an individual's personal decision, but I feel it is a decision that deserves to be made with a full grasp of all the facts and clear picture of the reality behind the illusion.

The adult industry is, in its most fundamental form, a fantasy factory. Whether a woman works as a webcammer, exotic dancer, escort, or porn actress, the goal is the same: selling an alternate reality. Craft an escapist world where anything goes, then make the audience believe the "magic."

Yet, most people have no idea what really goes on behind the veil. They have no grasp of how much this fiction costs performers as well as the audience. Nothing in life is free, not even free porn, and so what's the real price tag? What is the actual cost?

This book will reveal many secrets the industry doesn't want people to know because when we shine light into the darkness, the Trap loses its ability to leverage the shadows for its bottom line. Once exposed for what it really is, its hold loosens. At least, that is my hope.

What consenting adults choose to do in their private time is beyond the scope of this book. Regardless of anyone's personal opinions about the sex business or adult entertainment, I believe the public has a right to be informed. How do people end up in sex work? Why don't they leave? Why is porn viewership growing exponentially? Why are audiences demanding increasingly violent and depraved content? These are all very good questions that we will examine.

Before we break apart the Trap, why not begin with a simple and seemingly obvious question?

If porn is considered among the socially acceptable vices in many countries, why is there no warning label and only a sales pitch?

When Bad is Good

Adult entertainment in all its forms is essentially a product that is packaged and sold to a consumer. I would like to point out that it isn't unheard of for popular products to enjoy years of approval and even endorsement only to leave disaster in their wakes.

For instance, in the early days of cigarettes, ads touted how smoking not only made you seem suave and sexy, but better still, was good for you, too. Sounding familiar?

Seriously, google images of early cigarette ads.

Want to stay slender? Don't want to gain any extra weight while pregnant? Want to ease digestion? Smoke plenty of cigarettes. Tobacco companies also relied heavily on expert (i.e., physician) endorsements in early ad campaigns.

According to Becky Little's article "When Cigarette Companies Used Doctors to Push Smoking,":

> *R.J. Reynolds Tobacco Company created a Medical Relations Division and advertised it in medical journals. Reynolds began paying for research and then citing it in its ads like Philip Morris. In 1946, Reynolds launched an ad campaign with the slogan, 'More doctors smoke Camels than any other cigarette.' They'd solicited this 'finding' by giving doctors a free carton of Camel cigarettes, and then asking what brand they smoked.[3]*

The tobacco industry had its own stable of doctors ready to endorse all the wonderful benefits that came with lighting up. This was common practice until 1964 when the surgeon general officially published scientific reports detailing smoking's harmful and even deadly effects.[4] In spite of mounting evidence that tobacco consumption was directly responsible for a wide range of diseases, tobacco companies maintained that there was no clear proof their products were harmful.

It wasn't until 1998, after the tobacco industry lost a landmark class action lawsuit, that manufacturers were forced to disband the

Tobacco Institute and the Committee for Tobacco Research which had been formed and funded to disprove any negative findings.

Of course, these days, we would be horrified if anyone suggested that tobacco products were good for your health. How would you react if your doctor told you to take plenty of vitamins, eat lots of leafy greens, and make sure to smoke at least a half a pack of cigarettes a day? This seems absurd today, but, again, I'd like to point out that physician endorsements for cigarettes were common practice through most of the twentieth century.

Today, though, every tobacco product is legally required to print a highly visible surgeon general's warning label on all packaging. Not only that, but in the United States at least, the U.S. Food and Drug Administration (FDA) has levied such severe marketing and advertising restrictions on tobacco products that their marketing has all but vanished.[5] No more Joe Camel. No more Marlboro Man or Marlboro stock cars. No more Virginia Slims ads in women's magazines. Despite surgeon general warnings, however, people still smoke, dip, vape, and chew. It's an individual's choice. Only now, they are fully aware of the potential negative consequences. The choice is an educated one. Any marketing claims that tobacco products are healthy or even that they have less harmful side effects are now illegal.

Consumers still enjoy nicotine, because if nicotine didn't have any positive or enjoyable effects—delivering a dopamine rush, suppressing appetite, easing anxiety—no one would bother risking cancer. Yet, consumers are still given enough information to weigh the short-term zing of a cigarette or the calming effect of a smoke break against very real dangers like cancer, emphysema, etc.

The same argument can be made when we look at another popular consumer product: alcohol. Unlike smoking, there actually is research that demonstrates that moderate amounts of alcohol, particularly red wine, can be beneficial to our health. Alcohol consumption has been part of human culture since the dawn of civilization. Just like cigarettes, every bottle of alcohol sold today is legally required to list the most common negative effects.

As we go along, it is important to keep in mind that everyone is different, whether we are talking about nicotine, alcohol, or even porn. One person might smoke at a party and never touch another cigarette. Another can have a glass of wine a day with dinner and stop there. But these aren't the people most vulnerable to all the negative effects that can destroy careers and shatter lives. When consumed in moderation, alcohol doesn't necessarily present any serious health threat. The person who drinks only on rare occasions generally isn't likely to develop cirrhosis from alcohol. Even with tobacco, I believe we can all agree that someone who smokes ten cigarettes a year isn't excluded from risk, but also isn't necessarily at the top of a list of candidates for emphysema.

However, even the scientific community agrees that not everyone can moderate. There are those who, because of genetics, personality, or their upbringing, simply cannot stop at one drink. Some people pick up a cigarette after ten years of being smoke-free and are right back to a pack-a-day habit, or those people who are diagnosed with cancer but still can't stop smoking.

We don't ban these products, but we do treat them with the degree of respect due dangerous creatures. These substances are controlled and regulated, and we take great pains to make certain the consumer is not only of age, but also fully informed of potential dangers. On top of warnings for adults, federal and state laws have established legal consequences for selling tobacco products or alcohol to minors. Scientific research has led us to this point, but what about the science of porn? Yes, we are going there.

What About Porn?

Why do I mention cigarettes and alcohol? Because, generally speaking, if an adult wants to smoke a cigarette, have a beer, or watch a porn movie, it is nobody else's business. If our culture considers pornography a socially acceptable vice similar to tobacco and alcohol, then why doesn't the adult industry have to abide by similar rules and restrictions?

As consumers, we demanded legislation to make sure certain substances were off-limits to minors. We demanded warnings placed on cigarettes, alcohol, potentially addictive prescriptions, cough syrup, spray paint, glue, violent video games, etc. Anyone caught violating these laws faces consequences that range from fines to jail time.

Porn somehow gets a pass. Why? Most porn sites only require the potential viewer check a box promising they are over eighteen. Checking a box that promises the consumer is of legal age would be laughable anywhere else. Can you imagine a thirteen-year-old buying a bottle of vodka so long as he signed a piece of paper promising he was of legal age to purchase alcohol? Or a fifteen-year-old getting a job as a cocktail waitress because she checked a box on her application certifying she was old enough to serve liquor?

In the United States, eighteen-year-olds are old enough to pay taxes, vote, and even join the military and die for their country, but they are not legally old enough to buy beer. An eighteen-year-old actress is legally old enough to star in a violent gang bang film. Yet, the same teenage girl would be fined for possessing a pack of hard lemonade because she needs to be twenty-one.

If this all sounds absurd, it's because it is.

The fact that any minor with an internet connection can click on a porn site, check a box, and access millions of pornographic videos begs the question of why online porn companies are held to a completely different standard than all other companies selling age-restricted products?

How can the porn industry continue to shift the full burden onto parents and guardians but take zero responsibility for serving underage customers? Hell, even liquor delivery companies (hello, delightful pandemic services) make sure that the receipt is verified viva voce by both the delivery person and a scan of the recipient's government-issued identification.

As for the audience legally old enough to watch porn, the adult entertainment industry isn't required to display any warnings at all, which leads me to another unsettling question. If there is nothing to be concerned about, and porn poses no potential risks or dangers, then why is porn age-restricted in the first place?

Food for thought.

The Lines that Divide

It's no secret that people are deeply divided when it comes to their feelings about pornography. To me, the adult entertainment debate inevitably divides into absurd extremes, a clear us versus them, pro-porn versus anti-porn.

It's a war in which one group is always the obvious villain and the other the clear victim or righteous avenger. Since this book will explore the industry from all angles and in depth, I will simply say this:

> *What if both sides are right? What if both sides are wrong? What if the entire plan is to have everyone fighting? What if everyone realized they have been misled, fooled into a war where the only winners are those making billions preying on the most vulnerable, by which I mean performers as well as audiences.*

Because if both camps ever came together and realized that the Trap is actually designed to capture and use everyone, what might happen then? What might change?

With any luck, we might find out.

My Story

Before we begin our journey, it only makes sense for me to introduce myself a bit more formally. It's natural that you ask why you should listen to me, or, for that matter, trust me. Am I an unreliable narrator whose judgement and opinions are jaded by my own journey? These are fair questions, and I won't deny that I have opinions or that my experiences have had a profound impact on the way I see the world. However, this doesn't mean I can't analyze objectively or think critically. I hope my blend of anecdotal experience and leading scientific, technological, and sociological research will ease any of these misgivings. We do have to begin somewhere, and the beginning is the ideal place to start.

How did I go from a normal everyday person to porn star?

Growing up, I was square. Yes, I still use that word. *Square.* Dutiful daughter, theater nerd, and all-around good girl. Square.

I grew up in an abusive household. Maybe that is why I worked so hard to remain on the straight and narrow. If I was shiny and spotless, then perhaps outsiders wouldn't look closer and uncover the truth. Behind my family's polished Italian Catholic veneer, there was a lot of physical, emotional, and, yes, sexual abuse. My father passed away from cancer at the age of forty-eight. It was only after his death that the worst memories began to surface, memories of him molesting me.

Yet, to say my life growing up was all bad would be dishonest. We never went without, lived in a nice home, and wore nice clothes. I was active in drama and on stage. To the world, we were a completely normal family. There was no drinking, drugs, or alcohol. My family didn't have a ton of money, but we were safely middle class.

Being a good Italian Catholic girl, I married very young, and believe it or not, was still a virgin. I didn't have the first clue about boys, let alone sex. Nothing had ever been explained to me. What did I need to know about sex? My husband would teach me all that stuff, right?

My marriage was never exactly blissful, but it started out decently enough. My husband had a good job, and, though I worked retail, I dreamed of one day becoming a nurse. The change, like so many bad things in life, happened little by little. The first major sign something was terribly wrong was when our phone service was shut off. When I went digging through the bills, I noticed rows and rows of these "1-900" numbers. I had no idea what a 1-900 number was, only that it cost a small fortune every time he called one.

When I finally worked up the nerve to confront my husband about the calls, he told me he was searching for work out of state.

Those were long-distance charges. Eventually, when the "out-of-state" jobs didn't materialize, I stopped believing this story and called one of the numbers. Imagine my shock when I found out this was a *sex* line.

I couldn't wrap my head around him spending hundreds, even thousands, of dollars of his money—of our money—to talk dirty to strangers.

Anyway, I don't know what's different about my personality. Maybe I have a naturally curious and investigative mind, but I wanted to understand the appeal. Why would a man, my husband, be so drawn to talking about sex with strangers when he had me at home? I had already tried and tried the direct approach, only to run into a brick wall of lies every time. I needed another way to get to the truth, to the heart of the matter. So, I applied for a job with one of these 1-900 operations, and they hired me practically on the spot.

I worked for maybe a week talking to these men. The ladies in the office schooled me on all the things I legally could and couldn't say. We were all hanging out together laughing at these guys as we pretended to be anything they wanted—everything we certainly were not. All the while, the goal was simply to get their $5.99-a-minute by keeping them on the phone for as long as possible.

In a strange way, this experience offered me some peace. At first, when I had discovered that my husband had been sharing his deepest sexual desires over the phone with women other than me, I felt threatened to the core of my being. Voices careered through my mind, telling me I was pitiful, a fool. But once I participated on the other side of the charade and got to know the women behind the fantasy, I realized those voices were wrong. My husband was the fool.

After I came to understand the first-hand workings of the 1-900 lines, I again naively thought confronting him with the truth might save our marriage. If I could only make him see that he was trading his real wife who loved him for a fiction spun by grifters who only wanted his $5.99-a-minute, that he would stop. I tried to get through to him, to help him see it was all an illusion, to accept that they were average women who were using him.

Obviously, it didn't work and certainly didn't fix the problem. But, at least, it gave me some closure. I knew the women on those late-night commercials with the sultry voices really weren't long-legged beauty queens lying around in skimpy lingerie longing to seduce strange men to satisfy their nymphomania.

Nope, they were regular gals with stretch marks and scrunchies, their deep sexy purr usually the result of a pack-a-day smoking habit more than anything. It was a business, an act, a performance and nothing more.

Sadly, though, nothing I said could chip away at the fantasy's lies enough to crack through his delusion. Not long after I uncovered the 1-900 habit, I started finding more and more evidence of the appalling level of my husband's obsession. He had porn movies and magazines seemingly hidden everywhere. They always featured women who were the exact opposite of me, women who were bleached blondes with giant DDD boobs or larger.

Me? I think after my first kid I maybe went down to a negative A cup. Back then, two strategically placed mosquito bites might have been considered a breast enlargement. And here I was, up against all these women who had these giant, perfect, beautiful breasts. Questions kept circling around endlessly in my mind. *Why didn't he want me? What was wrong with me? Could I change? If I did, would he then finally have eyes only for me? Would he then be faithful to me and only me?*

Desperate for my husband's affection, I had my first boob job, but the surgeons could only make me into a C cup. Unsurprisingly, the breast augmentation didn't help. Shocking, I know. My husband's addiction to porn only worsened while my self-esteem plummeted. I was a failure. The one man who had pledged to love and treasure me, and only me, didn't. Far from it, as no matter what I did or how hard I tried, I was never enough.

By this time, I was working two jobs, frantically trying to keep up with the bills because his obsession with porn was devouring our finances faster than our marriage. This all came to a head when my husband got fired from his job. The how and why of his firing made my humiliation complete. Even now, I can't think about this time in my life without shame burning through me, even though I have nothing to be ashamed about. I was collateral damage. Sadly, though, what the mind understands the heart often refuses to believe. My husband had been fired for downloading thousands and thousands of porn videos onto the company's computers.

This all happened right around Christmas. We had a newborn baby at home, our first child, and I just lost it. It wasn't like I could leave him and go home. Even if my family would take me in, which I doubted, the shame was too much. I was alone and scared. Worse, I was trapped financially.

I needed to support myself, but even working two jobs wasn't enough to make ends meet. Something inside me shifted...or maybe just finally snapped.

If You Can't Beat 'em, Join 'em

Isn't that the old saying?

Since I didn't have a lot of options and was desperate to make money, I auditioned at a well-known local strip club. I got really drunk right before my tryout. This was totally out of character for me because I didn't drink and came from a family that didn't drink.

Alcohol was the only way I would have enough courage to go through with my plan. I needed to dull my "square" Italian Catholic values, silence my prudish upbringing, and muffle all the shame and guilt. That alone was enough to drive me to the brink of death by alcohol poisoning. But I managed. Besides, it isn't like I was the first girl to audition totally smashed, and, sadly, I wasn't the last. I was about to do a lot of things that were out of character, so what did it matter if I took up drinking? It sure as hell beat robbing banks. I got the job and resigned myself to my hopefully-temporary fate.

Obviously, money was the biggest reason I even considered being an exotic dancer, though not the only reason. I had so many emotions boiling inside me. Anger. *How could my husband do this to me? Our baby?* Revenge. *If he doesn't want me, I'll show him that plenty of other men do.*

While I had my fair share of dreams, growing up to be a stripper sure wasn't one of them. I had never been a promiscuous person. Even my brief stint as a 1-900 operator hadn't changed that. But I had already gotten my implants and saw a way to move forward, make a good living, and, at least in my mind, regain some power.

Power, of course, being money.

The club hired me practically the same day, and soon I was making far more there than I did working two retail jobs. It wasn't long before I was making enough to support myself and my son, meaning I was finally in a position to file for divorce and break free of a relationship that had been wrecking me for far too long. I had been stuck in this marriage for seven hellish years and now, at long last, I had a way out.

I wasn't exactly young when I started working in adult entertainment, which is highly unusual. I was maybe twenty-seven or twenty-eight. Though I was technically older than the other strippers, my parents had sheltered me to the point of a childlike naïveté that didn't change much with marriage. I knew nothing of the world beyond the simple boundaries of wife, mother, daughter, and reliable retail worker.

I was completely unprepared for the crazy world I had stepped into and had no clue what sort of predators I would encounter. In fact, it would take many years for me to appreciate fully just how evil the adult industry could be, and worse, how insidiously depraved it would become.

But I'm getting ahead of myself. Back to the strip club.

When I auditioned, my only focus was getting hired and making fast cash. I had no idea what the job would actually entail. Boy, was I in for a rude awakening. The job description said nothing about the fact that that I would spend only a fraction of my shift dancing on stage. In fact, the stage was a very small slice of the overall job. No, most of the time, I would be working the floor, hustling for tips, selling lap dances, and pushing drink sales to horny men who were all much larger than me.

It didn't matter that I was tottering around on sky-high heels, wearing little more than a thong and a smile, scared half to death. My feelings didn't get a vote because my feelings didn't pay the bills. The only thing that mattered was the job, which seemed fairly simple, but was actually far from easy. I was there to create a fantasy, convincing as many customers as I could that they were interesting, funny, and desirable so they would keep buying drinks and shelling out cash tips.

Sometimes, I entertained large groups: bachelor parties, crowds of rowdy college guys, or large tables of businessmen blowing off steam. Working a group meant a lot more money, but it also meant a lot more risk: more drinking, more testosterone, more personalities to manage, more stress. Drunks could go from laughing to throwing chairs, glasses, and punches without warning, possibly hospitalizing me before a bouncer could intervene. Constant vigilance meant higher anxiety, and higher anxiety meant drinking more to stay calm enough to remain in character.

Though in the beginning I hadn't fully grasped all that exotic dancing would demand, I was a quick study. Customers weren't my only constituency. Happy customers meant happy managers. Any girl who wanted promotion had to understand that happy managers were the real ticket to the premium shifts where cash flowed faster than booze. Hungry for the best nights that came with the high-end customers, I soon worked my way to the top, the place where a dancer could finally work smarter not harder.

By that point, I was drinking more than ever. Checking out in a boozy buzz made my job easier, the lies smoother, and my acting more convincing. Better still, the shifts seemed to fly by. The problem was that checking out might have seemed like a good emotional survival strategy, it was always a gamble with staying vigilant over my physical survival. Like all gambles, eventually my luck ran out.

One night, I went to an after-party. I had already drunk too much on shift, and just in general, I had grown too comfortable, too confident. Long story short, someone drugged my drink, and I was raped.

The rape destroyed me.

Before that terrible night, it was one thing to strip, let guys see me naked, or do lap dances because I was in control. It was a performance, not me. After being raped, everything changed.

When I returned to the club the following day, even the other girls realized something about me had changed. Any self-esteem or respect I had ever held for myself was gone. I could no longer dismiss all the awful things my verbally and emotionally abusive parents and husband had said about me for years, the names they had called me. They were right.

I was trash.

I was also angrier than ever, mostly at myself. How could I be so stupid? It wasn't as if I didn't know how common it was for dancers to be sexually assaulted. Anyone with an ounce of sense would have known it was always a matter of time before something bad would happen. Yet, I went and ignored all the danger signs and somehow thought the worst would never happen to me. That I could act so foolishly, believing I was somehow different or special, was unforgivable to me.

A short time later, when a group of porn stars and their producers and directors visited the club and offered me entry into their popular production company, I accepted. Porn paid a lot more money than exotic dancing, and the pay was far more reliable. Why not make the jump? In my mind, I was already damaged goods, already suffering constantly. I didn't believe it could get any worse. It was just higher pay for the same pain.

How wrong I was. While the money was a lot better, yet again, I didn't have a clue about what I had actually signed up for. A producer drugged and raped my friend and me, almost killing us both. So, yes, I was raped a second time. I don't know which was the worst. Being raped a second time, feeling as if I was too dumb to live, or the fact that nothing happened to the man who assaulted us. It ended up one of those "blame the victim" situations. Somehow, there's this ugly notion that any woman who consents to porn automatically removes her option to ever say no to sex.

What do you call a rape victim? A porn star who didn't get paid.

After what I had endured, I was irredeemable. I was no longer a person. I was a product, a commodity. I gained an agent at the expense of my agency.

There was no way to turn back time and make different choices, no way to undo being raped twice. I had a young son to take care of, so falling apart wasn't an option. There seemed only one logical path forward if I was to survive.

Make it to the top.

I had always possessed a solid work ethic with anything I did, whether that was being in drama, working retail, or now becoming a brand name in the adult industry. Along the way, I have done it all, from exotic dancing, to being in print as a *Penthouse* Pet, to webcamming, to performing in more than five hundred adult films.

In spite of my extensive body of work and the breadth of my experiences, I never stopped dreaming of somehow leaving adult entertainment. More than anything, I wanted a safe, sane, regular, boring life. As a mother, I longed to have a job that was acceptable for career day. I wanted to fit in and be "respectable."

Why didn't I just up and walk away? This is where it gets complicated.

Sex work has always been able to trap performers. In my experience, most women work in adult entertainment because of the money. Money, however, is more than a sum printed on a bank statement. Financial security is personal empowerment. Anyone who has ever had their credit card declined or an ATM machine spit out an insufficient funds slip can appreciate how much power a bank balance has. For the adult entertainer, money often represents a kind of control and self-determination that may have been previously absent. Money is a safety net that means we can take care of ourselves and don't have to beg for handouts or explain every penny we spend.

Also, as we will discuss in upcoming chapters, while this work has its perks, those come at a very high emotional, physical, and psychological cost. Entertainers can end up trapped because they grow accustomed to a certain level of lifestyle that is not easily replicated. Many remain because of addictions or because the business has damaged them so much that going back to being "normal" is no longer doable.

Like I said, I certainly didn't grow up dreaming of becoming a porn star, and most of the other performers didn't either. There are circumstances and motives and desperation we can all relate to, moments when life's hairpin turns that push us into corners or even off cliffs. Divorced mothers or single young women are trying to pay for education or earn enough to escape abusive situations. The fact the roulette ball lands on porn instead of XYZ option is all that separates the respectable struggle from degraded desperation.

There is a difference, though, from being trapped and being caught in the Trap. Being trapped is an anxiety-riddled perception and feeling, but the reality is that there are still options and choices. The Trap is something entirely different. It isn't a feeling or impression. The Trap is an entirely new reality and not a nice one: it's a nightmare.

On the surface, the Trap appears somewhat harmless, merely a twenty-first century way of delivering adult entertainment to twenty-first century viewers over twenty-first century devices. It appears to be just an updated version of the porn industry we have always known. If customers prefer to use a computer or smartphone instead of buying a paper magazine or video cassette, it only makes sense to change tactics. It's just good business sense, and unless the porn industry wanted the same fate as Tower Records or Blockbuster, it had to evolve.

And evolve it did.

No one in the early days of the World Wide Web could have predicted how ubiquitous, pervasive, and transformational the digital world would become.

In order to fully understand the Trap, we are going to explore all its component parts. How does it work? How does the Trap lure its target, and what happens when the target is caught? The first part of this book covers the performers and what really goes on inside the industry. In the second half of the book, we will step through the screen to look at how the Trap affects the viewers and consumers of porn.

Fair warning, the deeper we get in our understanding of the Trap, the emotionally darker and more culturally treacherous the terrain becomes. But I promised to be honest, and now, I am making another promise: no matter how dark it gets, there will be a light at the end of the tunnel.

Not Every Story is My Story

I'm here to share my experiences, what I have been through, and to speak truthfully about my years in the business. Yet, it would be unfair and inaccurate for me to portray every performer as a powerless victim or every porn viewer as a depraved misogynist.

We will be mostly be covering mainstream adult entertainment, not underground illegal sex trafficking or prostitution. While it might be an inconvenient and definitely uncomfortable truth, the adult industry historically has offered women the high pay, flexibility, and freedom that few other occupations could provide.

If I am claiming truth-sayer here, then here is another fact: while adult entertainment is mostly appealing to young, low-skilled workers with limited options, there are also educated professionals who deliberately choose to get into the field. It is narrow-minded and short-sighted to pigeonhole all adult entertainers into a dumb bubble gum-snapping Hollywood stereotype.

Over the years, I have known women who worked in adult entertainment to finance advanced education, pay off debt, supplement positions in professional careers, build up a nest egg, or simply have money for the niceties they couldn't afford with their regular nine-to-five jobs. There are even couples who perform together. They view working in the adult business as simply that: business.

Some enjoy the work and all the extras it provides from higher pay and flexible schedule, to doting clients willing to pay their bills, lavish them with expensive gifts, or even be there the way no one else ever has, such as footing the bill for an emergency surgery or providing a top-notch attorney when a loved one gets in trouble. The perks are as varied as the performer, but they do exist and are powerful enough to keep entertainers enmeshed in a life many know they should leave but can't find the way or the will. For me to portray all adult entertainers or porn consumers as identical groupings of people with identical motivations, desires, and experiences would not only be inaccurate, but it would also be insulting.

There has never been a universal type to do or consume porn, and that is especially true these days.

As I write this, our world has endured more than a year of the COVID-19 pandemic, with no clear end in sight. Our world has changed in ways we could never have imagined, leaving all of us a little uncertain, a little depressed, and longing for a little more human connection. It shouldn't be a surprise to anyone that stress, isolation, and anxiety have driven porn viewership through the roof.

If that wasn't enough, quarantines, shutdowns, lockdowns, layoffs, and furloughs have had a massive impact on all industries, including adult entertainment. People have lost jobs or had to close businesses, and plenty have watched their income go from comfortable to nothing. Savings only go so far, and not everyone who lost their job qualified for what little government aid was available. Some people haven't had a paycheck in months.

Regardless, these everyday people still have to feed their families, keep the lights on, pay the rent or mortgage, and make the car payments. As a result, tens of thousands have turned to adult entertainment as an accessible means—or, perhaps, a last-ditch effort—to survive the crisis. Many are starting to learn the hard way what they really signed up for, but, again, we will get to that discussion.

All in all, it doesn't and shouldn't matter why a person turns to adult entertainment, either for consumption or employment. What matters is what happens once they are entangled together on both sides of the screen or want to leave.

At the end of the day, though, for such a complex topic, it all boils down to something fairly simple: You don't know you're in a trap until you try and break free.

2

THE BAIT

The Trap is simple. The best ones usually are. Though I will refer to many different types of traps as we go along, I believe carnivorous plants offer the best introduction to the Trap for a few reasons: they blend into their surroundings, pretend to be something they aren't, and make promises they have no intention of keeping.

For instance, the Venus flytrap has, instead of an open bloom, an open mouth of petals lined with tendrils. Each tendril has a shiny glob of sugary fluids that dangles like candy. It all looks innocent enough. Look closer, and only then can you see there are tiny hairs all along the petals. The hairs are triggers waiting for the signal to strike.

The plant is primed and ready to snap shut at the right moment. Once closed, there is no escape, and the plant then slowly dissolves its victim alive.

Then, there is the pitcher plant, a climbing vine with leaves that form a bowl-shaped container. The bowl's edges are brightly colored, and its lips ooze sweet nectar. Color and the smell of something tasty are enough to lure in curious and hungry prey.

It is only once the trusting victim takes the bait that it realizes the sides are extremely slippery. Once the meal falls inside, it quickly learns there is no way out. The more it struggles, the deeper it sinks into the pool of digestive enzymes at the bottom where it will drown, die, and be absorbed, providing a feast for the predator who could claim it was really the prey's fault for giving in to temptation.

With the Venus flytrap, the pitcher plant, and the many other varieties of meat-eating plants, the story is the same. The prey spied something bright, sweet, and easy. The bait isn't just sweet, but it's also seemingly the necessary nutrients to sustain life. The prey only ventured close for a quick meal, never for a second suspecting that it was the meal all along.

I find a twisted sense of poetry in this because the Trap works in much the same way when recruiting, or luring in, potential performers: offer something essential, tempting, and seemingly harmless, then wait.

A pitcher plant doesn't catch every fly that whizzes past. The Venus flytrap doesn't clamp down on every bug that lands on its leaves. That would waste energy, and the plant would die. Trust me, the Trap hasn't thrived the way it has over the past two decades by wasting energy. Like these carnivorous plants, the Trap of our modern age prefers to hunt passively, offering what people believe they want or need, and promising them they can have it with ease. It disguises itself as an equitable partnership, dripping with choice, even oozing empowerment.

Regular plants offer up tasty treats as well. Their flowers freely feed hummingbirds and honeybees because that bird or bee will then zoom over to another flower and pollinate it, ensuring the plants will thrive. Without the birds and bees, the plants would eventually die. The bees benefit because they feed on the pollen and then use what they have gathered to construct honeycombs, make honey that feeds their queen and the young, and all this benefits the hive. Without the plant's flowers, and the pollen, the bees would die. This relationship goes both ways, but like all good relationships, it requires hard work, honesty, and real equality

Everyone wins.

With a carnivorous plant, only the plant wins. The bee is duped, doomed, then consumed.

Same with the Trap. Only the Trap wins.

Money Bait

The nectar for humans, more often than not, is money. Hey, it has always worked, why change? In fact, this bait actually works better in the modern age because so much adult entertainment is virtual, and thus can be done online, the internet providing the channel for cash flow via subscriptions, private performances, tips, etc. Also, the assumed anonymity of the internet makes people bolder, willing to take risks they might never have considered otherwise.

What did Pornhub's Dr. Betito say? Anyone can be a porn star!

You don't need any experience, require very little equipment, and can do it all on your own time. Work as much or as little as you want. No one needs to know, and, best of all, you can leave any time. If that isn't a sweet deal, what is?

There have always been plenty of desperate single moms, struggling students, and people tired of working three part-time jobs just to get by. The global pandemic has brought us double-digit unemployment, shuttered record numbers of small businesses, and rendered certain industries completely extinct. Suffice it to say, there are more than enough frightened people willing to override their better judgement for a short-term solution to very real and present problems.

The Trap has always offered plenty of promises. Once you get through school, out of debt, or on your feet, you can simply move on. The pandemic has merely added in new assurances of being just a temporary measure, a limited-time safety net. Once your job furlough ends and the company calls you back...once the pandemic restrictions lift and you can return to your old profession...once all that federal support comes in, then, you just walk away.

Or not.

We will talk more about the fine print later.

Beauty Bait

Granted, the lure of high pay is strong all on its own, but not everyone who takes the bait is desperate to feed their families or pay rent before being evicted. The Trap has been using this bait for years, long before COVID-19. Remember, money is always more than money. It is power, reinvention, and a way to rise above one's current status. The prettier the face, the more doors tend to open.

In our social media-saturated world, money can mean a whole new you, literally. And a whole new you, a new you that commands attention, respect, and leads to new and more lucrative opportunities, doesn't come cheap.

It is important to understand how the Trap is using our culture for its advantage. Females have always struggled with accepting the worth of their self-image compared to print and screen iconography, but the digital age has distorted reality to such a degree that low self-esteem has reached epidemic (dare I say, pandemic) proportions. In our selfie-centered world, we have become obsessed with the superficial. Is it still reality once in sepia?

Plastic surgery, hair and eyelash extensions, and fake tans are the norm. Our culture is addicted to filters and fillers, and why wouldn't it be? Think of all the reality television. A whole generation has been struggling to keep up with the Kardashians when they can't even keep up with themselves.

While men once dialed 1-900 and paid $5.99 a minute for one kind of fantasy, anyone with a smartphone can now pay $5.99 a month for an illusion of their own with some clicks and a few swipes across a screen. Even middle school girls are using special apps to make their noses thinner, lips bigger, ears smaller, eyes larger, on and on. We are bombarded with absurd pop culture standards that all relay the same message: *No matter what you are, you **are not** something else.*

If a female is naturally thin, then she will be ridiculed about her flat butt, stick legs, and flat chest. Legitimate complaints about her issues are taken as humble brags, and there are always the whispers about eating disorders. If she is busty, she will endure taunts about her "udders," mocked for being a cow, or labeled a slut because, you know, large breasts automatically make a woman promiscuous. If she is curvy, she will hear nonstop mockery about her "thunder thighs," and "horse legs," and probably deal with more than her fair share of bullying about being fat.

In 2019, the beauty industry raked in more than $532 billion dollars just for profits generated just in cosmetics and body care products.[1] These companies don't make this kind of money convincing females they are perfect as they are.

For years, we blamed the airbrushed models depicting unrealistic body types for the rising rates of body dysmorphic disorder (BDD) in teenagers and women. BDD is a mental illness defined by an obsessive fixation on a real or perceived flaw in appearance. A relatively new trend, referred to as Snapchat dysmorphia,[2] has many surgeons wondering if people are losing their ability to distinguish reality from social media.

Seemingly out of nowhere, patients started reaching out to plastic surgeons for procedures that could make them look like their retouched selfies posted on social media sites like Snapchat and Instagram. What doctors have found particularly troubling is that, while filters can smooth out skin imperfections or make a person's lashes longer, they can also alter an image to cartoonish perfection or reshape a face to alien dimensions.

It is one thing to request laser resurfacing for smoother skin with an even tone. But to completely alter the actual shape, symmetry, and dimensions of a face, that is an entirely different order and order of magnitude, and, sadly, an increasingly more common one.

In recent years, young men are also being diagnosed with BDD in record numbers. What was once considered a predominantly female mental disorder has crossed the traditional gender barrier and is now impacting males—younger males in particular—with devastating consequences.

Men are vulnerable to the beauty bait, too. Gym memberships, trainers, tans, stylish haircuts, and plastic surgery all cost money. A lot of money. Men have always been measured by how much they earn or the status of their occupation. This has not changed and most likely never will until our biological reproductive drive to seek out the best mate is eradicated from our brains.

Men are bombarded with unrealistic body standards deceptively proffered as normal. Images of men sporting chiseled bodies, six-pack or eight-pack abs, and strong, cut facial features grace magazines, websites, and ads. Of course, males also fail to appreciate that the flawless male models are the product of professional lighting and advanced software.

Graphic artists use programs to remove any imperfections, add muscle size, trim excess bulk, and layer in shading to craft the illusion of a perfectly defined physique. Computers transform a fit male model into action figure, editing away his humanity and replacing it with a caricature's dimensions.

Why am I taking the time to mention how pop culture warps body image? Because this phenomenon creates insecurities, shame, and self-loathing. The Trap uses insecurities, shame, and self-loathing for fuel. The negative pop culture impact crosses all barriers: gender, age, ethnicity, rich, poor, educated, etc. Everyone is vulnerable. No one wants or likes to believe they are unwanted or undesirable.

And if the solution to all your problems isn't within your budget? The Trap has the solution. Money alone is no longer the bait; rather, it's what money can supposedly do. Far faster than that plain old day job, the money offered by the Trap can supposedly transform your attractiveness, desirability, and self-worth.

Approval Bait

While men are obviously susceptible to beauty bait, that tends to work better on women. Men have always wrestled with self-esteem tied to wealth, power, and status. Now, thanks to ever-changing and increasingly unreachable social norms, the bar has been set even farther out of reach. Spend enough time on social media, and it's easy to believe that every guy but you is a baller. They all are C-level executives, own a Harley, wear designer threads, and have supermodel girlfriends with naturally enormous boobs whom they take on exotic vacations. The wife's Kindle is full of billionaire romances. It seems as if every woman at work talks non-stop about *Fifty Shades of Grey*, even though actual men who are any shade of grey aren't alive. They don't sit on a board, rather they lie in a coffin. But what does logic have to do with anything?

Want to be the guy with the custom suits who drives fast cars and attracts faster women? Offer a fiction.

Approval bait is particularly powerful. We all want to be admired, to be wanted, to even be envied. The Trap conveniently offers a shortcut. The Trap flourishes in our superficial consumer culture because so many people are desperately insecure. They are constantly comparing themselves, their stuff, their address, their lives with everyone else, even with people they don't know.

Even with people who aren't real.

How many home channels feature regular houses where regular people would live? That would be dull. Even house hunting programs can be absurd. Follow the early thirty-something couple on their search for a home within their half-million-dollar budget, which is a suspiciously high number for a postal worker and his wife who teaches pottery at the community center. Or watch the people who can only afford $60 thousand dollars to renovate a bathroom. Even movies and television shows portray a warped idea of the typical middle-class home. It's hard not to feel like a loser when we are bombarded with realistically unattainable extremes presented as normal goals.

On top of that, people of all ages scroll through their social media feeds and streams daily. They see friends who live in nicer neighborhoods, drive luxury cars, send their kids to private schools, and on and on. Snapchat dysmorphia might be an indication that we have lost touch with how real people look, but our social media and modern cultural myopia demonstrates that it's easy to forget how real people live.

We see curated lives, cropped and filtered into a fiction where we never quite measure up. The Trap thrives on envy.

3

THE TRIGGER

The Trap uses all kinds of bait, but not everyone is going to bite. Sometimes, the Trap has to study its prey, try different tactics, and wait for the right timing. The key takeaway about triggers is we all experience them at some point. We are all vulnerable, lost, hurting, overwhelmed, and broken at some point.

A person might have ignored the bait or not even noticed it a month ago, even six months ago. Then, something changes, forcing the person to make quick, emotional decisions.

The Trap is indifferent to our crises, external or internal. It has no conscience, only a sense for useful versus not useful, and that is what should really terrify us. The Trap doesn't care because it can't care, it can only sort.

The External Crisis Trigger

This trigger works best on those facing a life crisis they believe can be easily fixed with extra income. Simple. They need more money. These people don't have a fallback, escape, or any real system of support. Very often, more money really is the solution.

Maybe it's covering the rent, repairing a car, or paying off debt.

Perhaps the household income has taken a major hit due to a divorce, job loss, death, illness, or caring for additional family members such as an aging parent or grandparent.

Perhaps your roommate ghosted you without paying rent or their share of the bills? Did that longtime boyfriend empty your accounts, max out all your credit cards then dump you? Perhaps you just found out your stepdad gambled away your college tuition money, and now you can't pay for next semester. It could be your ex won't pay child-support, and your mom can't watch the baby, so you have to quit school. Is alimony no longer coming in? Maybe Social Security can't cover the bills after an extra cold winter?

Social Security? Yes, women of all ages are doing porn. More on that in a bit.

Whatever the crisis, it's a big enough problem that the prey is primed to make decisions out of panic. Money might not buy happiness, but it can buy a new transmission, cover a hospital bill, and keep you from having to drop out of college.

Triggers widen the holes that allow compromise and bargaining to start taking hold.

The Internal Crisis Trigger

There doesn't always need to be some immediate disaster for someone to be desperate, to be having a crisis of the soul. Earlier, I mentioned women usually end up in the adult entertainment industry because of the money. But, again, notice it isn't so much the money as what the money provides.

The Trap doesn't waste its time trying to catch those who are in solid relationships, who have a high self-esteem and a healthy group of close friends and family. Those who have that sort of safety net in place, by definition, aren't prey. Those who enjoy sound financial and emotional support and have a high self-esteem aren't hungry for any nectar the Trap could offer.

Toss in the right crisis, though. Eventually everyone is hungry for something, even if it's internal or emotional.

She could be anyone, from any social class. She could be driven to the breaking point by a controlling boyfriend, abusive husband, or her toxic family. She is always having to manipulate, plead, bargain, or apologize for what she needs or wants. Everyone and everything else come before her.

Nothing she asks for comes without guilt, no gift without strings. For her, money is freedom. Freedom to have something nice all for herself without needing permission, without having to beg. Her partner thinks nothing of spending their entire tax return, hers included, on a new motorcycle, a bigger flatscreen or a boat without any discussion. Meanwhile, she can't even buy a drugstore lipstick without handing over that pound of flesh.

She might seem to have it all to those seeing her on the outside. But, make no mistake, she has serious issues with low self-esteem, and believes she is only useful to those around her for how much they can take. Slowly, accepting a side job in adult entertainment starts looking like a practical way to have some form of agency and independence. She can call the shots for a change. Or she could finance fixing the outside because she has no idea what to do with the rotting mess on the inside. The Trap offers liberation, keys to nice things she wants, and maybe even a way to regain some power and dignity.

It doesn't matter what the story is. There is always some raw and aching need, a crack that can be exploited. Eventually, the internal void will expand until there's nothing left to fill it with except what the Trap can provide. Welcome to being useful.

The Life-Altering Event

The external or internal crisis doesn't need to be sudden. Some crises gestate over long periods of time. A life-altering event differs from the other two triggers in that it is always a shock. This trigger works on those who have always been relatively stable, then something yanked the metaphorical rug out from under their feet. It's something the person could never see coming, never really plan for. This can be an unexpected divorce, a betrayal, abandonment, heath crisis, rape, date rape, bullying, a sudden pandemic, or anything that renders the target completely exposed. Life-altering events are also ideal triggers because that is when external and internal crises join forces.

We have talked a lot about young people and social media. No, the Trap isn't some sentient creature lurking in dark corners of Instagram or Snapchat (or whatever happens to be popular), trolling for performers. The Trap isn't skulking around TikTok. While the Trap might not be a living organism like the Venus flytrap, that doesn't mean it doesn't have programmed directives to suit its need to continue to grow and thrive. To do this, what it needs, like the Venus flytrap, are good, reliable triggers.

The Trap, in this instance, might be better thought of like a computer virus. A computer virus isn't an organic creature, yet certain types of malicious coding behave so similarly the term *virus* is the most apropos. Just like a computer virus doesn't care if the recipient clicks on a corrupted link intentionally or accidentally so long as the end user clicks, likewise, the Trap isn't entirely particular what type of trauma makes a certain trigger work so long as it works. But, to continue the analogy with the computer virus, it isn't enough that an end user clicks, what is optimal is the target remains unaware that anything is wrong so the virus can slip in and wreak as much havoc, extract as much of the target resource (data, money, etc.) as possible without detection for as long as possible. The same applies to the Trap. It appreciates that online trauma often works just as well as real-world trauma, if not better. This is because shame, disgrace, or suffering can be made public or even go viral, and there is little to nothing the victim can do until it's too late.

Whether it's someone targeted by online bullying or, after a relationship sours, having their most intimate moments uploaded for all to see, the Trap doesn't care how the psychic breach occurs so long as there is a nice opening where it can slip in undetected. Whenever a person experiences something akin to having an A-bomb dropped their life, this is when the triggers are most likely to be effective.

What happens isn't as important as how impotent the person

feels, how mentally distracted and emotionally vulnerable they are. Maybe they have lived in a virtual world, leaning on relationships that don't exist. When the bottom falls out, how many of those hundreds or thousands of friends, fans, and followers really are going to be there? Like be there, be there. When reeling from trauma, it's easier to step on a trigger when one doesn't have others there to truly watch your back, in person.

First of all, let's imagine we are dealing with something particularly shameful like a rape. Definitely a life altering, life shattering event. What college coed is going to post those details in her feed? She is wrecked, damaged, and nothing will ever be the same.

What if, for some reason, she had to drop out of college? Lost a scholarship? Lost a small business? Everyone in life and online admires her. Most people aren't eager to announce failure to the world. She will do everything she can to keep that secret. Not to mention she will probably do her best to keep up appearances for as long as she can. This isn't exactly rare. How many people have lost a job and never told their spouse and pretended to keep going to work every day?

There are many who will choose to suffer in silence, struggling every day to find a solution on their own, terrified of being found out. Why? Because we live in a curated world where everything is cropped, edited, filtered, and perfect.

But say this person does open up about her small business going bankrupt or that her house just went into foreclosure. How will all those friends and followers respond?

Oh, they will send thoughts and prayers and healing vibes, but how many are going to wire money, pay her bills, offer angel investment, land her a job interview, give her a place to live, or offer something, anything meaningful?

Maybe it could happen, but probably not.

That's the problem with creating a fantasy life based on the illusion of friends. Friends—actual friends—have skin in the game. They are there in real life to help when everything falls apart. But even in real life, those friends are rare.

Too many young people have no concept how vulnerable they truly are until life sucker punches them. Bloodied, stunned, and flat on the ground, reality shifts into sharp relief. It becomes painfully clear they didn't have nearly as many friends as they believed; that they were always, in fact, alone.

The digital age's impact on relationships isn't limited to only young people, either. As we have become more and more connected online, we have become more disconnected in real-life. We've increasingly become a culture of "busy," believing that virtual friendships are as good as the real thing.

Now with COVID-19, many of us are realizing how we so blindly and easily traded authenticity for illusion. Or, if we did maintain real-life friends, we are now cut off from them. They are struggling just as much if not more than we are. The places we have historically looked to for support (i.e., church, support groups, friend groups) are off-limits. A lot of people are only now fully feeling how truly alone they really are now that so much we took for granted has been taken away.

It might be comforting to believe that only the young, the damaged and abused, or those living a high-risk lifestyle are teetering on the edge of ending up in adult entertainment. But never underestimate pride, which is just shame in a designer dress.

The Trap, as you will see in the coming chapters, is an omnivore. The people we idolize, whom our culture admires, have a long way to fall from such a high pedestal. The people who seemingly have the most to lose frequently don't and can't ask for help because they can't bear humiliation. If all they have left is what other people believe—the fiction that they are better or more successful or perfect or have it all together—they will cling onto that false narrative as long as they can even when they are emotionally bleeding out. It's human nature. There is no age limit on who the Trap denotes as useful. No social class is immune.

Today's Super Mom on Facebook might very well end up tomorrow's porn star. Keep in mind that, when her husband left her for another woman, she lost her small business, or was laid off from that high-paying job, she lost more than money. She lost her identity.

Everyone believed she had it all together. Look at her Instagram! And, until recently? She did. She made the right choices, worked her tail off, but it didn't matter.

Whether male, female, young, old or in between, these people all share something in common. Their comfortable lives just hit an iceberg and are sinking fast. Faced with a bleak and uncertain future, they are suddenly open to any solution they believe can keep them going until they get back on their feet.

Before the trigger, whoever has been eyeing that bait a little too long has not yet made any life-altering decisions. They have only started thinking, considering, weighing options.

Plenty of people have the same triggers and walk away and never take the bait. But, for some? They grab hold of the first thing that resembles a life raft and drift across the Trap's threshold, never knowing there is no way back.

4

THE CLOSING DOOR

A huge reason I wanted to write this book is that too many people mistakenly believe that those who end up in the adult industry are somehow different. They couldn't possibly be like you or your neighbor or the people you know from college, work, or church. Adult entertainers aren't moms, hair stylists, or car mechanics, and they certainly aren't part of the PTA.

I've got some news.

There aren't any giant signs on the highway of life, no exit ramp that reads "LIFE TRAPPED IN PORN—TEN MILES AHEAD." The Trap uses the public's ignorance and Hollywood stereotypes to hide what it actually is...and what it actually profits from.

When the average person imagines the pathway to porn, it isn't uncommon for the public to conjure a tired Hollywood melodrama. They envision the naive young girl who attempts a singing, modeling, or acting career that never quite takes off. With big dreams but no street sense, she is now stranded and struggling to get by financially in a big city like Los Angeles or New York. She is only one pretty face out of tens of thousands of others. Over time, she starts lowering her expectations, taking any work that pays, simply to survive.

It is only a matter of time until she is preyed upon. Maybe it's a seedy producer or photographer who pulls a bait and switch. Or maybe it's that bad boyfriend who turns into her pimp. Broken, isolated, ashamed, she can't ever go home, so she ends up on the pole. Addictions help her cope and, before she knows it, she is on her knees, on her back, doing porn. Cue the sad-but-inspiring-contender-for-best-original-song-Oscar.

It all sounds like a bad movie, right? Wait, it is a bad movie, quite a few bad movies, actually.

The Trap wants people to believe the *Showgirls* idea of who ends up in the adult industry and how, because it makes it easier for the Trap to remain camouflaged.

There have been enough people who took this path to engender and fuel the stereotype. There are the broken, abused, and addicted, too. The problem, however, is these aren't the only people who end up in adult entertainment.

The Trap wants the public to keep believing these stories, because the best lies are always rooted in truth. How many people tempted by the bait, and hit with some trigger, believe they are somehow safe from danger because they don't fit the profile?

Too many who end up in adult entertainment have no way of knowing what they have signed up for: not the short-term traumas nor the long-term repercussions.

The Trap offers the appearance of control, freedom, privacy, and even total anonymity. It wants people who join ranks to believe they aren't like those people. They're in control and are choosing to step through the door. Entertainers can keep their public persona and private work completely separate. Besides, why tell anyone since it's temporary?

Maybe the door slams, or perhaps it closes without a soft little click. The closing door is marked at the moment when money starts changing hands.

No two stories or two paths into the adult industry are alike. In fact, there are so many pathways through this world, we couldn't possibly tour all of them. Most who set foot through the door are not only desperate, but they are also ready to believe whatever they need to in order to make it.

Though male performers suffer plenty, I am mainly focusing on how the adult industry impacts women, not only because I feel I can speak more authentically, but also because female sex workers disproportionately outnumber males. Let's examine some of the more common ways women get into porn, and how it then starts to spiral out of control.

No one—at least no one I know of—signs up on day one to do a gang bang flick with ten guys, a bondage film where they would be beaten half-senseless, or a video with double or triple anal, double-vaginal, or some combination of any of this.

This obviously happens because thousands, if not tens of thousands, of these films exist. It happens, but it usually doesn't happen overnight outside of a sex trafficking scenario.

We will begin with pre-COVID-19 porn, since due to the pandemic, most film sets have shut down. The Trap has actually benefited tremendously from the general quarantine. Porn has been one of the only booming businesses because the Trap simply opened new roads. But, trust me, once the crisis passes, those old pre-COVID-19 paths are going to still be there, freshly paved and widened.

With the emerging messaging that porn is harmless, positive, and awesome, I am concerned that the Trap will be more powerful than ever.

The Traditional Door to Porn

Obviously, there are the more commonly known entryways into porn, such as the one I took—being discovered by an agent or someone prominent in the adult industry while working as a stripper, dancer, bikini model, etc.

There is the guy or girl who started out with dreams of becoming a famous actor, singer, or star, who can't seem to catch a break. This is more or less a direct path straight from whatever the person happens to be doing—dancing, modeling, performing bit parts in movies—to performing for the first time on a porn set. With the digital age and all the changes since the pandemic, I would be bold enough to wager that these doors to porn have been abandoned. The Trap only mimics the traditional adult industry, even in recruiting.

For the sake of education, we will dial back time and tour the porn world pre-2020—how it recruited, operated, etc. We will assume that, once the lockdowns stop and the professional studios reopen, the adult industry will go back to business as usual.

As I already mentioned, porn can be a career, and a lucrative one at that. Though as you keep reading, you will see this career is brutal. But that's for later. For now, I will grant that if a gal is savvy and manages to end up with a decent agent, she will have a fighting chance to last a lot longer in the business and land the safer jobs with better pay.

As an example, for a girl who starts out young, around age eighteen, the industry will often play up the little girl or jailbait angle with school uniforms, pigtails, and bows in her hair. She can expect to begin with girl-girl, move on to girl-guy, then on to threesomes, and eventually into harder and rougher hardcore porn the longer she remains in the business.

If she creates a strong fan following and keeps halfway sober and sane, she will have a lot more ability to turn down jobs that are dangerous or would wreck her physically and mentally in a matter of months. She will be able to draw a line she won't cross because she will have a fanbase and their buying power that she can leverage.

As she "ages," she will go from playing jailbait babysitter at eighteen to the hot horny stepmom within a couple years at the ripe old age of twenty-three.

This sort of performer might last the longest, but she is rare, and trust me, she will get hurt. Pain, disease, exploitation, psychological and emotional trauma are part of the job. The female body isn't designed to endure the increasingly extreme boundaries the porn industry pushes to keep audiences hungry for more. Granted, most films are completed in a single day, but this single day consists of eight, twelve or sixteen hours where multiple partners subject a woman to every form of penetration, often including foreign objects, in every orifice. Depending on the script, she could be humiliated, bound, gagged, or even beaten. There are some production companies I refused to work with because of their reputation. I knew filming automatically came with a hospital stay afterwards. Actresses who had worked with them required weeks to heal enough to work again.

Tragically, too many girls get into the industry already too damaged and desperate, or too naive, and what the work demands costs them big time. They are quickly used up, their bodies ruined, and psyches destroyed. The Trap is a meat grinder and the performers don't matter.

There are too many pretty fresh young things who can replace her. As we will discuss in a later chapter, meat grinder girls, tragically, often end up performing in the remote realms of freak show porn that cater to every bizarre fetish imaginable.

The Digital Door to Porn

In the modern age, the Trap doesn't scout like it used to because it doesn't need to. With the internet, most prospects will actually come to them.

The indirect or digital path is now the increasingly common entree to the porn set.

A lot of work in adult entertainment can now be done online with a smartphone, tablet, or laptop. It can begin relatively innocuously with providing sexting chats, or even the modern VoIP version of a 1-900 number. This sex work "lite" then progresses into webcamming for the obvious reason that it means more money.

Webcamming holds a lot of appeal as a starting place because it can be done from home, a woman can work as little or as much as she wants, and there is potentially a lot of money to be made. The more skin you show, the more the cash flows. All you need to do webcamming is a computer, a place to do your job, and something to show that will attract and build an audience.

I could say a performer needs a young, hot, "bikini bod," but the truth is that audiences have a wide range of what they find appealing. There are women and men of all ages, shapes, and sizes performing via webcam.

While writing this book, I have read many articles that I found less than honest when describing this area of the industry, what is required—or even demanded— to make it. There may be a few new girls in this business who make money by doing very little. I haven't seen them, probably because they are the equivalent of a unicorn.

Despite that inconvenient reality, I have seen webcam work glamorized as a form of self-empowerment and entrepreneurship, which, technically, is true. Yet nowhere was there any mention of the high-risk nature of this job nor an accurate description of the physical and emotional costs.

True this is a business, but it's one fraught with danger, vulnerability, and an automatic and permanent stigma—the Scarlet XXX. Yes, permanent. We will unpack this phenomenon more as we go along, but this inability to ever leave and start a new life is one crucial difference between the adult industry of old and its new digital imposter, the Trap. Remember the missing warning labels we talked about in the beginning? The first on the list should be, "Once you are in you can never leave."

A new webcam performer might begin timid and showing only a bit of skin, but the false sense of privacy and the temptation to make more money eventually makes many of them bolder. In webcamming, the more extreme, dangerous, or degrading performances that entertainers are willing to offer, the more fans they will get, the more repeat business, the more subscribers or private clients, and this means more money.

Once the performer starts crossing the boundaries of their comfort zones and limits, the money comes in even faster. Keep turning the heat up and up and up. Go totally nude, add in sex toys, be willing to participate in violent, dehumanizing, or downright dangerous acts, such as autoerotic asphyxia (i.e., placing a plastic bag over your head), etc. The more a performer is willing to do, the more money hungry audiences are willing to pay. The problem, however, is the demand for increasingly extreme content will go up as well. There is a sharply rising number of viewers who get off watching women suffer and can only become aroused watching pain and humiliation. Webcamming clients can ask and are willing to pay extra for some crazy stuff, especially those who are turned on by violent acts against women. I once had a client who requested and paid to see me riddled with bullet holes and act as if I were dying. I wish I were making this up.

I used lipstick to cover myself in "bullet holes" and then flopped around like I was in my last convulsive death throes. The same guy kept hiring me, insisting I do this again and again. Guess my "dying" wasn't convincing enough for him to get off. Another potential customer requested a scenario where he wanted to see me, "get punched a million times in the stomach." Yeah, I turned that one down.

Over time, two things happen for webcammers: they become numb to the incremental shocks of crossing their personal boundaries, and they become accustomed to and dependent on the steady and increasing inflow of money. The consequences of this could take up another entire book, but here, I'll break it down into two broad categories of what could happen.

Those Who Consent

For the relatively new entertainer, what was once insane has become a new normal. They have acclimated. Why not go to the next level, from webcamming to actual porn on a set? Webcamming is time-intensive, hard on the body, and a constant hustle, whereas porn is comparably stabler. The only difference is the level of exposure, but often the entertainer has come to accept that she cannot remain hidden and make the premium pay simultaneously.

If clients can encourage the webcammers to cross boundary after boundary with private performances, it isn't uncommon for fans to also push webcam performers into doing films. There are those who decide that porn is the next logical step in their career. They have already gone this far.

They are high on the attention and money, and, so far, they have been able to maintain a strict separation between who they are in real life and their persona as a performer.

Someone who has been successfully webcamming knows there is a ton of competition. In order to outpace other performers all vying for the same clients, she needs to do more than just webcamming. She must make a name for herself and expand her fanbase. Porn films generate fans who then are willing to pay for webcamming and more. As a result, she seeks out an agent and books her first foray into an actual porn film.

What does it matter? She has grown accustomed to living a double life. There is the person everyone knows, then the fiction she has created behind closed doors.

She can easily explain a trip to Los Angeles or Las Vegas as vacation or even work, depending on what her regular job happens to be. While her first film seems like the ultimate line she never thought she'd cross, it's just the first in a set of lines that will make crossing webcamming boundaries look like a game of shuffleboard.

At the risk of sounding crass, there is a honeymoon phase when you are first in the business. You are making all this money, you feel important, you have a ton of attention. She has a false sense of anonymity and control. Who knows how long this ride will last? Might as well make as much as she can. For someone who is damaged or has been emotionally abandoned, it's a rush!

Besides, it isn't as if she is doing anything illegal, and no one needs to know, right? Wrong. This was what I meant earlier when I said the industry really doesn't need to go scouting like it used to. Performers come to them.

Those Who Cannot Consent

Then there is a darker side of how someone can go from webcamming to doing porn on set. First, there is always a risk that a client could be filming any performance from his side of the screen. Maybe the clients keep the footage to themselves, but they could just as easily upload it online later for their own personal financial gain at the expense of the performer's anonymity.

That's just a risk that goes with the job, but, for the record, not where I have witnessed the vast majority of webcamming-to-porn-set transitions occur. Just keep in mind it is a possibility.

As far as I know, most webcamming sites are not somehow in cahoots with clients. They aren't encouraging these customers to go around uploading essentially pirated videos because, for one reason, that is lost money. Secondly, it's too many unnecessary steps the companies don't need to take. They are a business and the private sessions are their particular bread and butter.

Where I have seen the change from webcamming to making movies, more often than not, happens when a girl realizes she has been duped.

There are plenty of shady webcamming companies who will assure a performer that the sessions between her and any clients are private, and streaming live, and are not recorded, when that is totally not the case. In reality, the company is secretly recording her performances, then selling them. She had agreed to perform private webcamming sessions, not unpaid erotic displays for global public access. Maybe this possibility—that the company could use content in any way they so choose forever and ever and in any medium currently in existence or yet to be invented in the future—was listed in the tortuous language of her absurdly convoluted contract. Maybe not. Like the terms of service we all click to simply move on and get what we need, the odds are better than good that the webcam company has every demand slanted wholly to their advantage. They know with 99 percent certainty that any potential entertainer isn't going to first hire their own attorney to slash through line by line and have those terms argued and adjusted before they go to work.

This is why, when the webcam company sells her performances, she is stuck, and they slide.

Besides, once she finds out, whom is she going to tell? How is she going to fight? If she fights, she only risks exposure when she has been doing everything possible to keep her two lives separate.

She never volunteered for this. She agreed to a private, tightly controlled environment with what she thought was a guaranteed degree of privacy and anonymity. Instead, a company knowingly took advantage and used superior knowledge, resources, and a massive power imbalance to extort another, weaker party and entrap them for the end purposes of financial gain. In short, she did not consent because, by definition, she couldn't consent. While she could legally argue they took unfair and unjust advantage, she won't. These companies count on her silence, appreciating that she will be unable to fight back without the battle costing her more than she could ever stand to win.

This is when our old friend reasoning stops by again. If she is already "in porn" anyway, then why not make the best of a bad situation and walk away with as much money, power, and status as possible? Why not at least get the upgrade in pay that can also give her an edge in other areas like webcamming?

In for a penny, in for a pound.

Pandemic Porn

I have tried to start this book so many times and for some reason or another, I never made it past a certain point. I admit this made me half-crazy not too long ago, but now, I can't help but wonder if the timing wasn't tragically perfect.

Since COVID-19, filming has shut down everywhere for all shows and movies, porn included. Strip clubs have closed. Strippers and escorts are out of work. It would be reasonable and logical to assume that the adult entertainment industry, like so many others, is taking a financial beating unlike anything it has ever known.

Or is it?

Certainly, some areas of adult entertainment have been, at least, temporarily shut down. But the Trap is actually stronger than ever because it discovered that it really only needs an internet connection.

The Devil is in the Data

Before we continue, I would like to refer to the most unbiased source possible...raw numbers. Though obviously we will talk about people, we can draw insights from analyzing the behaviors and choices people make.

In this case, the data alone reveals a stark truth hiding in plain sight.

Even before the pandemic, online porn sites were breaking all previous records, not only for how many people were watching porn, but for the staggering number of new contributors and amateur performers.

To keep this simple and brief, I will focus on probably the largest and most well-known adult entertainment site, Pornhub. Online porn was already growing exponentially before quarantines, lockdowns, and the emergence of entirely new groups of people desperate for work.

According to Pornhub's own end of year business report for 2018:

Now we're not saying that size matters, but 2018 was an impressively big year for Pornhub and its users. Visits to Pornhub totaled 33.5 billion over the course of 2018, an increase of 5 billion visits over 2017. That equates to a daily average of 92 million visitors and at the time of this writing, Pornhub's daily visits now exceed 100 million. To put that into perspective, that's as if the combined populations of Canada, Poland and Australia all visited Pornhub every day! [1]

Keep in mind, these numbers are directly from a major porn

outlet...and Pornhub is only ONE of many outlets. But wait, there's more. From the same report:

> *Pornhub's servers served up 30.3 billion searches, or 962 searches per second. To make sure there was always fresh content to satisfy those searches, Pornhub's amateurs, models and content partners uploaded an incredible 4.79 million new videos, creating over 1 million hours of new content to enjoy on the site. If you were to start watching 2018s videos after the Wright brother's first flight in 1903, you would still be watching them today 115 years later!* [2]

From a purely business and profit perspective, this is incredibly positive news. Their own infographic announced that there were 33.5 billion visits to Pornhub in 2018, with an average of 92 million visits daily. The site handled 30.3 billion searches at a staggering rate of 962 searches per second. In 2018, visitors uploaded 4,791,799 videos, which translates into a million hours, or 115 years of video.[3]

The infographic goes on to relay how in one year, there were 4,403 petabytes of data transferred, which works out to 574 MB of data for every person on the planet. In one single day, Pornhub visitors consumed more bandwidth than the entire internet used in 2002.[4]

When we look at Pornhub's year-end report for 2019, the steep rise in porn consumption is brain-melting:

> *Pornhub keeps on growing and it doesn't show signs of letting up. In 2019 there were over 42 billion visits to Pornhub, which means there was an average of 115 million visits per day. One-Hundred-Fifteen Million – that's the equivalent of the populations of Canada, Australia, Poland and the Netherlands all visiting in one day!* [5]

The increased number of viewers was the equivalent of adding another country. Pornhub boasted 39 billion searches for the year, which was 8.7 billion more than the previous year.[6] The company goes on to say:

In 2019 there was a record amount of video uploads, over 6.83 million new videos were uploaded to Pornhub. To put this in perspective—if you strung all of 2019's new video content together and started watching them way back in 1850, you'd still be watching them today![7]

In twelve months, Pornhub added the equivalent of 153 more years of video. The marked increase in viewers and added video are shocking enough, but this part of the article is what really caught my attention because it reveals a trend that they had no idea would explode in 2020:

Over 98,000 new models joined Pornhub, bringing the total number of verified models to more than 130,000! ...it may come as a surprise that 'Amateur' was the top of the list for 2019's searches that defined the year. Perhaps this was in part due to the incredible number of new verified amateur models that joined the site. [Emphasis added] [8]

If you check out the 2019 Pornhub infographics, the United States doesn't just lead the world in porn consumption, but we leave the other countries in the dust. Americans average 10 minutes and 36 seconds per visit.[9]

Keep in mind this was the average visit, at least for Americans before COVID-19. This was when Americans still had to go to work, attend classes, or could go to a mall, a movie, a bar, or even on a date. This was also before hundreds of millions of people were ordered to remain home, and millions were forced to find new ways to make money in all this so-called free time.

Can you imagine how that number must have grown in 2020, how many more visitors there were, how much longer the average visit became? Also, if 98,000 new models joined Pornhub in 2019, how many signed up over the course of a pandemic when millions have been furloughed, laid off, or had their jobs or businesses simply disappear?

However, we shouldn't expect the numbers for 2020 to provide us a direct apples-to-apples comparison, since Pornhub instituted sweeping changes in mid-December of 2020.

The company landed in hot water after a *New York Times* expose prompted Visa and Mastercard to cut ties with the porn giant.[10] Pornhub purged millions of videos, taking the number of videos on the website from 13.5 million videos down to slightly under 3 million. Pornhub promised to ban viewers from downloading content, increase the number of moderators, and pledged to permit only those who are verified—content partners or those part of their Model Program—to post content.[11]

While this is a promising move forward in policing and monitoring content to make sure the videos are legitimate, the acts consensual, and all participants of legal age, keep in mind that these changes were only instituted a couple of weeks before the end of 2020. How many more videos were uploaded, then downloaded by viewers before the changes? The videos among the 13.5 million removed by Pornhub aren't likely to vanish when either the creator or bootlegger—someone who downloaded a video previously uploaded by another person only to upload again—can simply keep uploading these videos on other sites that don't yet have the same restrictions.

Also, keep in mind that Pornhub is only one source of adult content, though it is one of the largest and most well-known. There are other sites out there that eagerly stepped in the gap for those unable to work during the pandemic. More specifically, certain sites have made it easier than ever to sign up for sex work and this has only fueled the unprecedented expansion of adult entertainment.

In March of 2020, Only Fans reported a 75 percent increase in overall new sign-ups — 3.7 million new accounts, with 60,000 of them being new creators.[12] According to Claire Downs' May 14, 2020, article in *Elle Magazine*, "OnlyFans, Influencers, and the Politics of Selling Nudes During a Pandemic,":

OnlyFans was launched in 2016 just as adult entertainers and sex workers were being shut out of platforms like Instagram, Patreon and Tumblr, thanks largely to the passage of the FOSTA—SESTA bills.

> *OnlyFans' loose content restrictions allow creators to put racy queued images and videos behind paywalls and engage with monthly subscribers through custom videos, DMs, and exclusive pay-per-view shows. Frequent payouts, and OnlyFans' comparably low 20 percent cut (most cam sites take 40 percent or higher), make the site incredibly popular.*[13]

FOSTA (Fight Online Sex Trafficking Act) and SESTA (Stop Enabling Sex Traffickers Act), which were passed in April of 2018 to combat illegal sex trafficking,[14] might have been well-intended. Reality, however, has since demonstrated that these acts have, in fact, had the opposite effect, actually making it harder for law enforcement officers to do their jobs and easier for sex traffickers to do theirs.[15]

The impact of FOSTA-SESTA alone is a hot topic all on its own. I only mention these acts because they have generated a ripple effect that has not only negatively affected professional adult entertainers, but it has also opened the floodgates for everyday people to step into sex work, mistakenly believing they can make fast and easy money.

The above article goes on to report that as of May 2020:

> *OnlyFans reported a 75 percent increase in signups, with 150,000 new users creating accounts daily.* [16]

Think about the numbers I just listed from Pornhub, and now add in the numbers from just *one* more site. How many of those 150,000 new users added *daily* can be counted on the roster of adult entertainers in 2020? Though we might not ever have the hard numbers, this doesn't mean we aren't already dealing with the collateral damage not only in the U.S., but also abroad.

They key takeaway here was simply to paint a clear picture of just how many people have been signing up to do sex work. Before COVID-19, porn certainly wasn't suffering from a dearth of those willing to work in adult entertainment. Yet, it appears the pandemic shifted this industry's expansion into hyperdrive.

Now that everyday people have been joining *en masse* simply to survive, the Trap will have an even greater impact than ever. Online content never goes away, ever. Once it's out there, it's immortal.

There comes a point you can be hit so hard, be down for so long, that a unique sort of desperation sets in, especially when taking care of the ones you love most. Of all people, I understand this all too well.

Previously held moral standards, beliefs, and social acceptability separate from part of your identity and become luxuries you can no longer afford. Before the pandemic, I feel like many among the general public intellectually understood this kind of despair. But now, the raw struggle to survive at any price has hit home and hit hard.

In this section, I have provided numbers and data, but what should be sobering to us all is that statistics have stories.

Facts have faces and families.

The Impact Area

COVID-19 has hit out planet like an asteroid strike. It has decimated small businesses and wiped out entire industries all over the world. Some of these industries may one day return, but we are all stuck in the meantime and the future is very uncertain. What is certain, however, is that the power company won't take a check from the Bank of Someday and trying one's best doesn't buy groceries.

The United States has a significant portion of their population that works in the service industry. This means when tourism, recreation, and all those "nonessential" industries were either shut down or so restricted that they have been operating on life support ever since.

Businesses shutter, jobs disappear, and families and individuals suffer.

Imagine any sporting event and how many jobs it creates, from the workers who prepare or clean the stadium to those selling merchandise or popcorn. Then, there are the businesses nearby, the hotels that once booked full during games, the restaurants, bars, clubs, etc.

When travel is shut down or restricted, this halts tourism, which impacts the airline industry. If tourists can't visit a beach, what happens to all those small shops that sold souvenirs, the stands that rented bikes, or those who made a living offering horse-drawn tours to visitors?

Casinos, amusement parks, the hospitality industry, and entertainment venues make up some of the largest employers. Recreation dollars are the lifeblood for many major cities such as Las Vegas, Orlando, and New Orleans, to name a few. The workers hardest hit by the pandemic are oddly labeled nonessential, but how long will places like Nevada last without their largest industry?

Some small towns have no other industry but tourism. How long can they hold on with no one skiing, hiking, climbing, diving, snorkeling, fishing, etc.?

It will be decades before the impact of COVID-19 on our economy can be accurately measured. But what happens when that tattoo artist, hair stylist, personal trainer, bartender, card dealer, hotel manager, tour guide, sommelier, or whatever suddenly has no income, and some don't even qualify for federal aid?

What, then?

I'll tell you what, then. The dark side starts seeming more like the bright side. I mentioned emerging sites like OnlyFans earlier. This is a site where you can do anything you want, even a cooking show. But there is a lot of steamy stuff on that site that requires no cooking range...unless you can create a fanbase willing to pay to watch some highly unconventional uses for kitchen utensils.

Invasion of the Amateur Performers

Everyday people are using their webcams and harnessing their assets because they have to get by. The problem is, like many short-sighted decisions and short-term solutions, a lot of those eagerly hopping online aren't aware of the Trap. They are acting out of survival instincts and are inexperienced in the industry which blinds them to the long game.

Though I certainly understand why they are turning to adult entertainment, I worry for them, too. They have no idea what they are actually getting into and possess little to no understanding of the long-term consequences this decision will have on their futures.

I know degreed professionals who have been laid off or let go. They are working to maintain an already expensive lifestyle. Before COVID-19, they might have even been living below their means until their businesses collapsed or jobs disappeared.

Then, there are the working class who were barely making it before all this mess. Now with OnlyFans? Webcamming? They might be making more money than they have ever made. Sure, they were desperate going in, but now that they are working in adult entertainment? They might be wondering what kept them from doing this for so long.

But notice I used the word "might." They might make excellent money. The problem, however, as I have mentioned time and again, is there's a never-before-seen glut in the market.

The Ripple Effect

The sudden and unforeseen surge in the number of new performers has also impacted a group you might not have thought about: entertainers who were already established in the adult industry.

Some of those who had been making an excellent income in adult entertainment are now struggling from shutdowns. Many webcammers who had transitioned into porn also worked in other areas of the industry such as stripping or escorting. Some also had jobs outside the industry that have been impacted.

My basic point is they had multiple streams of income.

But as social distancing, shutdowns, and closures have left performers stuck inside and going solo as it were, many are working harder and longer than ever for less and less pay. Audiences are feeling the financial pinch and aren't as free with money as they might have been before the crisis.

An April 2020, article in *Newsweek*, "Sex Workers Say Online

Market Is Saturated With Performers, Fans Are Canceling Subscriptions During Coronavirus Pandemic," reported on many of the unforeseen consequences that have rocked the adult industry since the shutdown. Unable to keep social distancing requirements, filming and production has come to a sudden stop and performers and crew sent home.[17]

This is a sucker punch in and of itself, but what many people don't know is that the application for the federal Small Business Association's Economic Injury Disaster Program clearly specifies that anyone who presents, "'live performances of a prurient sexual nature' or derives their income from 'the sale of products or services, or the presentation of any depictions or displays, of a prurient sexual nature,'" is ineligible for its support.[18]

Established online performers are losing customers or making less money because audiences are dealing with their own financial struggles. Before the pandemic, they might have been able to maintain a comfortable living and set strict boundaries. Now? To remain relevant, keep current customers and entice new ones, these entertainers have far less power to say no regarding the content they create.

A year and a half ago, they might have never considered performing autoerotic asphyxia. But these days, they are competing with hundreds of thousands of new content contributors who are also hungry. If they don't do it, someone hungrier will.

Some performers might work directly with individual customers through Discord, a chat app favored by video game players. There are many other platforms including Chaturbate, OnlyFans, and Skype, but again, the surge of new sites, combined with the crush of amateurs rushing to cash in, creates entirely new problems for anyone trying to scrape out a living.

The Darker Side to The Dark Side

First, with COVID-19, online platforms offering these sorts of services have experienced a skyrocketing number of subscriptions.

According to the April 10, 2020, article in the *New York Times*, "Sex Work Comes Home,":

Daryn Parker, the vice president of CamSoda, said there had been a 37 percent increase in new model sign-ups this March, compared to last March. For the same period, Bella French, the co-founder and CEO of ManyVids, another camming site, said that there was a 69 percent increase in new model sign-ups.[19]

This number has continued to grow at breakneck speed.

Women new to webcamming soon realize they are starting at an automatic disadvantage. Unlike a professional adult entertainer like myself, who simply moved over to OnlyFans to make do during the shutdowns, these new additions have no pre-existing brand. They aren't entering the arena with an established platform where they can recruit longtime fans directly to becoming subscribers. These women lack a key advantage that could help them be successful—the power of numbers.

Numbers—large numbers—are the only way to be successful on these sites, and it has to do with how these platforms pay. For instance, members pay an average of five dollars a month to view an OnlyFans account, with twenty percent of that fee going directly to the platform. There is an additional five percent commission subtracted if the performer was referred by another contributor.

A professional can count on automatically converting a portion of her fanbase and have hundreds of loyal subscribers almost immediately. She isn't starting from ground zero.

Most of the new performers can barely reach double-digits in subscribers. Being a nobody competing against thousands of other newbies to create a brand out of nowhere means that, to make money, they have to find ways to stand apart to be competitive.

Women have little choice but to perform more and more extreme acts to gain attention, quickly realizing the dirtier they get, the more subscribers they can retain and attract.

They are working around the clock, non-stop, as viewers grow more demanding about what they expect for that five-dollar subscription. Many performers soon face a hard truth they hadn't considered before. If they want to keep making money—enough to be considered making a living—they will have to give up their ability to set boundaries or say no. They are not in control of the content, not really. Virtual reality can quickly become a literal hell.

When I write, "working around the clock," this means hour after hour, day after day, shoving vibrators, dildos, and other foreign objects of all shapes and sizes from the tiny, to the bizarre, to the large and grotesque into their bodies . The physical toll, even physical damage, can be severe. Then add on the emotional and psychological strain, and that is a formula for a nervous breakdown, injury, or even accidental death.

According to the *BBC* article, "Hope Barden: Sex role-play death prompts law change plea,":

> *Hope Barden, 21, was found asphyxiated after carrying out a degrading sex act on the Internet for a pub landlord over 250 miles away.* [20]

Hope Barden, a young woman in the United Kingdom who had turned to webcamming to subsidize her income as a caregiver for the mentally challenged, died while the client on the other end watched as she begged for help, claiming she couldn't breathe. He didn't call for any emergency assistance, and Hope's body was discovered by a roommate two days after her death.[21]

Some women performing online during the pandemic were already in abusive relationships and are being coerced into this line of work either directly or indirectly. How many are living with an abusive partner who has the power to kick them to the curb if they don't bring in any money? There are new reports surfacing where women report being forced into webcamming then blackmailed with exposure if they don't continue.[22]

As if it couldn't get worse, the law offers little protection. For instance, according to a May 2020, article in the *Daily Record and Sunday Mail*, "Scots women warned sex webcamming is not easy way to make money during lockdown," journalist Annie Brown reported that:

> In March, a cache of stolen pornographic photos and videos from the subscription website OnlyFans leaked online. Scotland's 'revenge porn' laws on non-consensual sharing of sexual images doesn't cover material which has already been voluntarily made public. [23]

There are also plenty of documented cases that demonstrate the very real risk that a performer can unwittingly attract dangerous or violent stalkers or become a target for harassment or outright attacks. Additionally, some women who have turned to adult entertainment while on furlough have returned to the workplace and been let go because of the stigma associated with the industry.

The pandemic won't last forever, though what the future will look like is anyone's guess. Porn might go back to business as usual, though, like so many industries, probably with some changes. Even if that change is something as simple as film location, the show will go on. Trust me, I know what it is to do what you have to do to make it. But once the new normal emerges, even I can't say precisely what that will look like, only that porn isn't going away. This means there will always be demand for new porn entertainers, which means webcammers willing to make that next leap.

Any upgrade in pay comes at a heavy price. Even while webcamming, a performer might have to rely on alcohol, pills, or drugs to numb herself and drown out her conscience. It isn't easy to live a double life, constantly in fear of exposure. Psychological toll aside, the human body isn't designed for repeated trauma hour after hour, day after day, week after week and so on.

Again, the Trap benefits from the false belief that a performer only needs to go as far as she wants and can leave at any time. Performers have taken the bait, stepped through the door. With all the glitter and lights, or the stress and chaos, the performers hardly notice that, at some point, an invisible hand has turned the key.

5

THE LOCK

After a performer steps through the door but realizes it isn't what she signed up for or decides she would rather do something else, why doesn't she just leave? Just as there are no simple answers to why or how someone ends up working in the adult industry, there are no easy answers to why they don't leave.

In this chapter, we will address the concept of the lock. But, before I can hope to explain the lock, please keep in mind that the Trap is effective because it's so terribly complex. It's like trying to unravel a strangle-vine that has already been allowed to wrap and tangle itself everywhere.

The Trap is a new and invasive species determined to spread. While society, legislation, or protest groups busily exhaust themselves hacking away at what is above the surface— what can be seen —this does little to nothing to stop the Trap because the Trap doesn't exist in physical space.

This was why in the opening I made a distinction between the adult industry as we have always known it and the Trap. Brick-and-mortar venues such as strip clubs, adult shops, peep shows, tanning salons, massage parlors, escort services, adult bookstores, and movie rental stores have always been vulnerable. They could be shut down, constrained by new laws, or picketed until forced to close.

Then, the adult industry was handed the greatest gift it never could have imagined—the World Wide Web. The internet, an idea that ideas, images, video could be easily shared all over the world with the tapping of some keys, has stepped out of science fiction and into everyday life.

Pornography shifted into virtual, borderless worlds where any rules, restrictions or laws could be outmaneuvered or ignored with a click of a button. While this has made it easier for audiences to access pornographic entertainment, ostensibly with guaranteed privacy, it's also taken a toll on the performers. New technology means upgraded locks.

The lock can take on any number of forms.

The Financial Lock

It always seems to go right back to money, doesn't it? The financial lock is simple and effective. Our person-turned-performer entered through the door for a reason, and that reason almost always is about money and what it provides.

This might be freedom, safety, security, empowerment, crisis management, or even a way to provide for loved ones. Once the performer starts making money, however, her lifestyle and or ability to provide for others changes drastically.

She now can afford a nicer place to live, a car that doesn't constantly break down, better clothes, healthier food, and improved medical care. Money offers more options.

Our performer isn't stuck living in the only apartment she can afford, she can choose to buy a home in an area of her choice. She can relocate to a safer neighborhood where she isn't worried about being robbed every time she steps out to buy groceries.

If she has children, she has the means to make sure they can play outside, attend better schools, engage in extracurricular activities, and more. She no longer is forced to live with an abusive partner because she couldn't make it on her own, she can afford to leave, to move.

She might have crossed through the door alone in search of a better or safer life or to take care of loved ones. Now those dependents rely on her to keep providing at the same level, if not better.

The financial lock is the most basic way the Trap keeps performers from leaving. Though crude, it works brilliantly for the simple reason that the choices become much harder. Make thousands of dollars a day or week that pays for a nice house, good schools, a safe car, medical care and even some savings? Keep the freedom to work when and where and how long to work?

Or return to an honest job (likely more than one job), working forty-plus hours a week for a fraction of the pay? Accept a job with no medical or dental benefits? No paid time off? No vacation? No sick leave? No security? Go back to living hand-to-mouth hoping life will remain within the budget. Because returning to a regular job means leaving behind the financial cushion to soften or absorb financial blows.

Better not get sick or have anything break down.

No matter how much a performer might want to leave and go back to being "respectable," deep down, she is keenly aware that crises happen. People get sick, cars break down, and disasters can pounce from nowhere. In fact, the chances are more than good that the entire reason she stepped through the door in the first place was because the bottom dropped out from under her, and she blindly grabbed hold of what she believed was the best way out.

Or even her only way out.

Desperation is still burned in her mind, her memories and pain real and raw. She will do anything to avoid being helpless. At this point, if she is considering getting out, the internal struggle makes her hesitate and again, start reasoning.

She would be giving up a lot of freedom, control and power to gain what? If she wants to work a normal "respectable" job, that can mean returning to that rundown apartment, moving her kids back into the dangerous neighborhoods into the most poorly funded public schools, if not removing them from private schools.

Instead of being at home and, to some degree, an involved parent, she will have to work longer hours to make ends meet, returning her to the role of absentee parent. Once again, she will need to rely on others—daycare, after school care, friends, family, partners. She will once more have to depend on people who might not have been reliable before. Maybe she thinks how everyone will get to watch her kids grow up but her.

All this to be considered socially acceptable?

That is a lot to give up. She can walk away, and some do, or at least try. How many will bargain and compromise? How many will remain snared in a trap of their own making because they are already negotiating, bargaining, and reasoning? If she can continue under the radar, keep her secrets, she will be able to provide, and can leave at a better time.

The stakes are high, the risk is real, but the performer is gambling regardless which path she takes—leave or remain. Remember, most of the areas of adult entertainment we will be discussing in this book are not illegal. Even prostitution is legal in certain locales. Technically, she is not doing anything against any law, and this can be enough to make her put off her exit...and keep putting it off.

But the financial lock is only one of many.

The Emotional & Psychic Lock

Thus far, we have only scratched the surface of what happens when a person crosses the threshold of the door. For almost every person who ends up in adult entertainment, they entered with some sort of wound. Some kind of damage. Sure, we can make this about money, but not every person panicked to pay a bill turns to porn as a solution.

Certain people are more vulnerable.

Wounds power the trigger that sifts the damaged, broken, lonely, angry, and abandoned and ushers them through the door.

Tangled Webs

Let's use webcamming to start with since it is one of the most popular and fastest-growing areas in pornography and is often portrayed as the more harmless areas of the adult business.

That isn't exactly a lie. But it's not exactly the truth, either.

Let's start with what is true. Webcamming technically is safer. A girl isn't at a strip club where she can be attacked in a parking lot or followed home. She isn't physically on set where she can catch diseases, be abused, or end up on the wrong end of a bait-and-switch. She isn't an escort, where she is placing her safety and very life in danger with every appointment. She isn't beholden to a service to curate a client list and ensure she has enough "dates" to make money.

I have lost count how many pop culture articles I have read about webcamming, all packed with interesting anecdotes and opinions. But you know what I have not seen? The truth.

The ugly truth.

Webcamming might appear safe and easy, but trust me when I say you can never unsee what is on the other side of that screen.

Private webcamming sessions are particularly appealing because they offer a sense of anonymity. Private sessions can even pay better because the entertainer is catering to the needs of one particular client.

The human mind may resemble a supercomputer in many ways. However, it doesn't come equipped with a trash can where we can drag and drop shameful memories then click delete. We can't update to fix trauma bugs and can't reset to factory settings to just forget these things ever happened.

Make no mistake: just because the interaction is virtual, it doesn't mean the performer is completely safe.

Keep in mind that the entertainer can *see* what happens on the other side of her screen. What's even worse? She is only half of this perilous game and has little to no control over what transpires on the client's end. No control over what images might end up seared into her mind.

No matter what I've done in front of the camera, some of the most deranged, depraved, and horrifying acts I have ever seen were from the other side—my side—of a webcam session. From men humping their pillows and inserting everything from X to Z into themselves, to having sex with blow-up dolls. I have inadvertently witnessed drug deals and even bestiality. Over the years, I have encountered fetishes I wouldn't have believed existed until I saw them with my own eyes.

And I can never not see them.

The webcam performer can't stop remembering what she has been asked to do during those hours, the roles she has played, the words she has said or that have been said to her.

There is also a physical toll, because many clients are paying to watch a performer masturbate, use sex toys, insert giant dildos, vibrators, or other foreign objects into their bodies, and to do so with a passionate enthusiasm designed to convince the client he is the only man she has seen that day—or ever, for that matter.

Repeat this same performance hour after hour, day after day, and who wants to sit on anything but an ice bag, let alone engage in real sexual relations with a partner or spouse?

This relentless mental and physical onslaught, over time, can't help but change a person. You have to harden, layer on emotional armor and compartmentalize because it's the only way to keep doing the work and not lose your mind.

When articles mention webcam performers, "working twelve hours a day," I feel they too often report this as emotionless fact. The words, "working twelve hours or more a day," are stated as if it's no more meaningful than mentioning there is a 20 percent chance of rain today

I ask you to envision what is really happening during those twelve hours. The webcam performer is engaging with those who, to the outside, appear to be ordinary or even respected men at the basest of levels. Many are fathers, grandfathers, husbands, professionals, or even community or spiritual leaders. They are masturbating, cross-dressing, telling the webcammer all their darkest and dirtiest desires. While many fantasies are far from criminal, it doesn't matter. Over time, the onslaught cannot help but skew and often jade her perception of all men.

At least it did for me. I started to think of every sexual interaction as being one-sided. Intellectually, I understood it was business, but emotionally, it was all take, take, take. What could the other party take from me? What would I have to watch and pretend to enjoy? This created a hard shell that walled in a lot of anger, as I imagine happens to other performers.

There is an illusion of control, but that control shatters especially when some fantasies cross into the horrifying, disgusting, taboo, or even outright criminal. If the performer wants to make money and keep her job, she has to play along and make the client believe she is turned on, too.

She risks ending up wrapped into fantasies of rape, incest, sexual acts with a minor, kidnapping, torture, bestiality, necrophilia, etc. Clients are coaching her, in great detail, telling her precisely how to act out their most depraved needs for their pleasure.

All the while, she is watching seemingly ordinary people at their weakest, worst, and in extreme cases, most terrifying. On some level, she accepts she is feeding these desires, crafting and fulfilling the most repulsive reveries.

Maybe she dresses in knee socks and school uniforms and, with bows in her hair, plays the part of the innocent schoolgirl the client longs to rape. Or, like me, she covers herself in fake bullet holes and blood. She then gasps and thrashes about because some guy is willing to pay big money for the thrill of watching a woman suffer and die because it's the only thing that excites him.

Obviously, there are more examples, but pretty certain I have made my point.

How can these interactions not eventually poison her thought life? Taint her opinions of others? Destroy her opinions about men?

Or of fellow human beings? Just as she is being dehumanized by others, she, in turn, must dehumanize them as well.

They are a paycheck, not a person.

Her lens, how she sees everyone, including herself, warps and distorts. She is stuck in a web she has helped weave, and guilt, shame, and disgust cling to her. She bears their shame as well as her own.

The Isolation Lock

What can entertainers do to minimize damage? On the other side— her side—of the screen she can master the art of disassociation as a protective measure.

Before we delve deeper, I would like to define what I mean by dissociation. Dissociation is a break in how the mind processes information. It's a state where you disconnect from thoughts, emotions, memories, and sometimes even your environment. In extreme forms, dissociation can alter the person's sense of identity and disrupt even the basic perception of time.[1]

The practice of mental dissociation is a common survival mechanism. Those who enter into the adult industry from abusive backgrounds are often familiar with this tactic. Victims isolate their being from traumatic experiences like being molested, raped, or abused.

Someone new to the business, however, might be completely unprepared for what they are about to witness. They lack the emotional armor and mental safeguards of those who joined ranks already battle-hardened from abuse.

Disassociation is common practice in all areas of adult entertainment. Even when I was doing porn films, my body might have been on set, going through the motions, but my mind was shopping or re-organizing the garage. To the viewing audience, it appeared I was having an incredible sexual experience, relishing every moment of carnal pleasure. In truth, my physical self might have been present to film the scenes, to do my job. But the inner me had already left the building and was somewhere far away.

While disassociation can somewhat protect the entertainer from one type of damage, unplugging over and over comes at a cost.

Think of yanking out a power cord from a USB charger. The first so many times you can get away with it. The connection works fine. But keep yanking that cord, and soon you have to jiggle it or fiddle with the angle to get the two ends to work together. Do this enough times, and soon the cord/charger connection is too damaged. When you try to plug it back in, you get nothing.

This is what happens when a performer keeps having to divide her physical body and her core self over and over.

You separate your body and spirit so many times that eventually they no longer fit back together the way they once did. Eventually, they might no longer fit together at all. The self is now locked in a state of perpetual isolation.

The feeling of nothingness becomes the new normal. Over time, the ability to form meaningful emotional bonds becomes too damaged and is eventually lost. The disassociation that kept the performer from falling apart served its purpose, yet it remains ingrained even should a performer no longer need its help. Even though she is safe to be once again "plugged in," she can't and thus loses out on some of the most rewarding aspects of her humanity and what others have to offer.

Humans are, by nature, social creatures. We need relationships with others to remain mentally healthy. Relationships require vulnerability, and for many, letting anyone in is no longer an option. There is too much shame, guilt, resentment, anger, and regret. Our performer no longer trusts anyone, no longer believes she is worthy of any kind of love, not even friendship.

Many who entered this line of work had no support network or a weak one. They have also gone to great lengths to keep their work in the adult industry separate and hidden from others, thus they have been leading double lives. Balancing two identities is easier to do alone. The fewer people to face, to lie to, to keep secrets from, the better. Steadily, the performer self-isolates more and more.

After a certain amount of time in adult entertainment, everyone is painted with the poisoned brush, and the performer is "damaged goods" in more ways than one.

Then there can be added complications because, while these jobs aren't technically illegal, there is the constant worry of exposure. Think of being a parent and trying to support a child, but then risking that child learning how Mom puts food on the table.

Guilt and shame compound.

The Addiction Lock

The entertainer is broken, alone and emotionally and psychically flayed. To continue to perform, she must cope, compartmentalize and disassociate. Eventually, many can't do this without some sort of a substance to help. To keep working, many adult entertainers have to rely on drugs and alcohol.

This drags the person deeper into the jaws of the Trap because addictions cost money. Addictions fool you into believing you are coping, that you are "fine." Pain is necessary because it's a natural signal that something is wrong. Pain keeps us from touching hot stoves, alerts us we stepped on a nail, signals when we have twisted an ankle or torn a muscle and should stop moving until we tend the injury.

Removing pain might provide a superficial benefit, but at what price?

Some passed through the door because of an existing addiction. Others develop the addiction once inside. The substances could be completely legal, like alcohol or prescription medications, or combinations of both. Some of the most effective drugs for treating anxiety also present extreme risk for addiction and abuse, Xanax being a good example.[2]

A lot of performers find themselves strapped to the see-saw of anxiety and depression, the dips and dives growing higher and lower. Then maybe they can't sleep, so add in some sleeping pills.

If girls can end up dead webcamming, they can also be seriously injured, too. The job might appear simple enough, but the performer's body isn't designed to endure constant trauma. Pain pills, anyone?

Back when I was shooting porn movies, I injured my back filming. Scenes can and do go horribly wrong. My arm, shoulder and fingers started going numb and eventually I needed back surgery. After that surgery, I slipped four disks in my neck and had to have surgery again. I was okay weaning off pain pills after my first surgery, but after the second? The addiction lock got a stranglehold on me. Instead of taking time to completely heal, I did webcamming to keep my income flowing since I wasn't ready to go back on set.

Webcamming was easier than ever. I no longer had to rely on sheer force of will to disconnect, because the powerful narcotics made it easier to check out. But just because I had managed to deaden my mind, didn't mean the damage suddenly stopped.

That would be like injecting your hand with lidocaine and resting your palm on a stovetop. Maybe you wouldn't feel the burn, your hand slowly cooking, but the flesh would tell a very different story than the mind.

Eventually, for the love of my family and with their unwavering support, I was able to overcome the addiction to pain pills, but sadly, there are many who are not so fortunate.

Of course, there is always the lure of illegal drugs as well. Male and female performers take uppers to stay thin, keep working, and be high and happy. Amphetamines for a boost, and barbiturates to settle down. The addiction lock can keep one comfortably numb, tucked inside a safe, warm place and no longer caring, no longer recalling there was ever any other way to live. Drugs, used to cope and mentally endure, can even become part of the fuel that keeps the spiral going. In a twisted irony, many performers start out needing drugs to do the work, only ending up needing more work to do the drugs. Back and forth, round and round and down and down.

Though I have only mentioned a few, the lock can take on count-less forms, and most people stuck in the Trap are held by more than one. The Trap counts on redundancy, knowing that money, shame, guilt, isolation, and addiction all work together to keep the performer in her place. She might wriggle free of the financial lock, but then she has to pick the psychological lock, break the of the isolation lock, and cut the addiction lock.

Some figure out the combination and break free, but in my experience, they are rare. Most resign themselves to their fate, which brings us to the next layer of the Trap.

6

THE CAGE

At this point, the performer might realize the door is not just closed, but locked. Life has taken a dramatic shift. She is no longer in control and soon realizes the work that was supposed to give her freedom, financial liberation, the ability to do as she wanted when she wanted, is a lie. She is now in the cage.

What's worse is that it is largely a cage of her own making. Society even says it's a cage of her own choosing.

Why did I choose to talk about the lock before the cage? Because whenever a performer steps across that blurry threshold, it might be clear she has entered a new realm. But too many naive souls still possess this skewed perception that they can simply retrace their steps and go back out the way they came in if they don't like the work.

While many would-be performers might grasp how their world will change externally, few have the slightest concept of how they will transform on the inside. They underestimate the Trap's corrosive power and believe themselves immune, the exception. That is, until the damage is done.

The hellish, hidden nature of this cage lies not in the entertainer being walled off in some dark oubliette. Rather, the bars of her cage allow plenty of daylight, even visitors. She can see the world outside, filled with normal people leading normal lives, but she is no longer like them.

We have already talked about all a performer would have to give up if she leaves adult entertainment. There are unforeseen problems, too. What is she going to put on that job application or resume to explain that gap in time and professional job experience? Can she pass a background check?

She might end up caged in webcamming because someone, maybe an abusive partner or angry ex, knows her secret and threatens her with exposure. Many webcam companies also engage in shady business practices and count on desperate people either not reading the fine print or failing to fully grasp the impact of the fine print.

When a webcamming company dictates that it owns all the content, this means they can re-sell that content, and distribute it any way they want for as long as they want. This means some webcam performers can unwittingly end up trapped in porn. Companies record her sessions then later upload that content to RedTube, Pornhub, or other adult sites. Though the webcammer never signed up for that level of exposure, she has little-to-no recourse if a company repurposes her performances.

Also, as we will explore in an upcoming chapter, even a brief presence in online adult entertainment will immediately create permanent digital links that, once fashioned together, become chains she will never escape.

Thus far, we have focused a lot on webcamming, but that is only one job among many in the adult entertainment industry. I am going to give you a tour of other areas of the industry, how they work, and how they cross-pollinate.

The Stripper Cage

Strippers have a well-deserved reputation for earning excellent money. Like most jobs in adult entertainment, the exotic dancer's cage can be financial. Also, like the webcam worker, porn star, or escort, she will have a tough time explaining the gap in her work history.

However, the stripper cage is unique in that the longer the dancer remains in this particular profession, the more she depreciates in value. Like a car, only with a beating heart, dreams, and a soul.

This area of the adult entertainment industry demands a certain level of beauty, youth, and fitness. Unlike a webcammer who can cater to any number of viewer tastes with her performance, or use tricks of lighting, angles, and background to maximize assets and minimize flaws, the exotic dancer has no such luxuries.

Granted, some dancers have a good head on their shoulders and accept they have a brief shelf life. They save or invest their earnings or use that fast cash to put themselves through some sort of schooling. These women prepare for the future. They capitalize on the high pay and minimal work hours to set up an exit strategy from stripping from day one. When they leave stripping, they will have a profession waiting and can practically wipe out or even erase any student debt. Some might funnel earnings into the stock market, buy up rental properties, or save enough to have seed money for starting a business once they hang up their thongs.

These aren't the type of women who will end up trapped in the stripper cage because they go in with a plan and a healthy respect for danger. They view exotic dancing strictly as a business. These women use stripping and don't let stripping use them.

Of course, these dancers are rare. Remember, most of the women who end up as exotic dancers were already damaged or desperate enough to even consider this sort of work. They have been exploited their entire lives, so exploitation is as common as air.

Some might get into exotic dancing with the best of intentions, like using the money to pay for a degree. But then their environment changes them, and their dreams become just that. Dreams. Far too many dancers spend money as fast or faster than they make it. They adjust their tastes and lifestyles to a level where they are living paycheck-to-paycheck. Tragically, though, they are in a profession where good money will be increasingly harder to make.

Many strippers cage themselves with poor planning, failing to save or invest in doing anything else. Sadly, the months or years a girl spends dancing not only make her less valuable in stripping, but without any schooling, training, or plan, the outside world won't have much to offer.

She might be fit for menial employment, entry level positions, or tip-based work in the service industry, but not one of these jobs will pay remotely close to what she has grown used to. Though the actual numbers will vary by club, the area of the country, and the establishment, even a day girl at a C-list club is likely to make more than even the best paid hourly retail worker (and largely in cash).

In my experience, the top dancers in the premium clubs can rake in six figures working only two to three days a week. These women forge connections with powerful, rich men who can and do open doors of opportunity. They can even form friendships. Clients frequently pay living expenses, provide cars, vacations, and lavish their favorite dancers with gifts, beauty treatments, plastic surgery, personal training, and spa days. Strange as it might seem, a devoted customer might even be one of the few people a dancer can count on to stand in the gap for the unexpected, like picking up the bill for a medical emergency or purchasing a last-minute plane ticket so she can visit a sick relative.

A stripper doesn't have to be among the lead dancers in Vegas for clients to serve as a by proxy support system. Maybe she works at a run-of-the-mill club in a blue-collar town. This doesn't mean her best customers might not pay her overdue rent, fix her car when it breaks down, or perform a badly-needed root canal for free because they genuinely want to help her somewhere other than the club. Sure, it's a dysfunctional support system, but it might be the only one she has.

Strippers have to consider some of the same trade-offs as the webcammer if they want to leave and seek more socially acceptable employment. She will be giving up being paid higher than her skillset would command anywhere else, but by now, I hope it's clear it isn't only money. She will also have to walk away from the partying lifestyle so ingrained in her work that she is likely dealing with addiction. Drinking cocktails all day is generally frowned upon in most other lines of work. When she leaves, customers who acted as a safety net will quickly move on and "be there" for another dancer.

Time is not the stripper's friend, but the sweet pay and fringe benefits are enough to make many dancers hang on as long as they can. However, the longer they hang on, the more secure the cage becomes.

The nature of how this realm of adult entertainment operates can become a cage all of its own, with dancers fighting their way to the top, then doing all they can to stay there. It's easy to get lost, for the world to fall away and grow smaller, the club consuming everything as days become weeks, months, and then years.

How does this happen?

There is a hierarchy in the stripping world, a distinct difference between what is referred to in the business as Day Girls and Night Girls. A club isn't going to waste the hottest and fittest dancers in their stable on midday and midweek shifts.

Day Girls staff the slower times where, while the club might be open, audiences are comparably sparse. A Day Girl is at a marked disadvantage compared to a Night Girl. She isn't considered the top talent to begin with, so that already works against her.

Then, day audiences have to get back to the job. They don't have the luxury of time that night clients enjoy. The Day Girl doesn't have much time to build rapport and hustle for extras. It's much harder to push drink sales to men who have to drive back to the office or have to at least appear sober in a meeting.

Day Girls have to work much harder, and the tips are not only tougher to earn, but they are slim pickings compared to what Night Girls earn during the club's premium hours of operation. The competition to earn slots at night and during peak hours where the booze and money flows freest is fierce.

Strippers have to keep watch over their face and figure, or they risk losing the best shifts, best days, or even their jobs. Beauty and fitness are a dancer's currency. They could potentially earn a dancer a top spot as a Night Girl from the outset.

Or should she improve her physique and invest in her looks, she can quickly promote from Day Girl status up to Night Girl. She might even work her way to increasingly more prestigious clubs. Beginning as a Day Girl then with plastic surgery, extensions, etc., she can keep working her way up to Night Girl.

Exotic dancers frequently invest in breast augmentation, butt implants, nose jobs, and a long laundry list of other plastic surgeries to outdo the competition and earn the best days and shifts. Not only that, but with enough upgrades, a dancer could possibly earn a spot at one of the more distinguished clubs that cater to only high-end clientele such as professional athletes, celebrities, lawyers, stockbrokers, etc.

Artificial body enhancements are necessary for those seeking an edge, as well as for those who want to extend how long they are able to keep earning the excellent pay they have grown used to.

Sadly, these investments end up being a double-edged sword. The physical modifications that work in their favor in the world of stripping are the same changes that could keep them caged.

While looking like sex-on-legs is a tremendous asset for a dancer on stage, it becomes a very real deficit off-stage, both in everyday life and after leaving the profession. Unless a stripper is willing to go back under the knife and endure the pain and expense to have the most obvious changes reversed—such as having large breast implants removed—the dancer's appearance alone can make it hard, if not impossible, to blend in effectively and be taken seriously outside the world of adult entertainment.

People love quippy sayings like how we shouldn't judge a book by its cover, but that's a bunch of bull. Humans judge solely off appearances all the time. It's in our nature, hard-wired into our brains through biology and evolution.

Consider that strippers work clubs within commuting distance. Every time she shows up to perform, she has to hope and pray that a coworker, client, or customer doesn't recognize her from the club and out her.

Should she try to find a different job, employers most likely to overlook the gaps in work history and lack of relevant or professional skills are frequently hiring her for her looks. They have plenty of positions she can fill, most of them not listed in the job requirements. I went through this many times, myself. The first time was right after earning my nursing degree. I naively believed my worst days were behind me and I could start anew. Though I was a skilled and capable medical professional, it never took long before my boss or other men at my place of work, even doctors, were cornering me, making lewd comments, propositioning me, or even trying to follow me home.

Anyone else could run to human resources, but me? Blowing the whistle would only bring unwanted attention to my unrelated thus undisclosed work history. Then it would be game over. Didn't you know that exotic dancers deserve to be felt up, propositioned, and sexually harassed? Sarcasm aside, it really was always just a matter of time until I was let go or finally had to leave because of stress or safety concerns. I am not alone. This is reality for the stripper trying to leave her cage.

Eventually, the dancer reasons that if she is going to spend an entire shift being sexually harassed and treated like a slut, why not do this all for a hell of a lot more money? And while buzzed from drinks she doesn't have to buy?

She is in a lose-lose situation. Those employers most willing to hire a pretty girl with a thin work history and an iffy background often have an alternate agenda. Employers who require a robust resume, long list of verified references, letters of recommendations, and that perform thorough background checks on all hires are probably safer workplaces that wouldn't tolerate sexual harassment. The kick in the tail, however, is the employer that would protect her the most wouldn't even consider her as a viable applicant.

Too many workplaces are reluctant to hire a woman who might prove "too distracting" to the men. She might also create a source of gossip, friction, and hostility among the female coworkers. Management understands that workplaces are already cauldrons of drama as it is, so why would they knowingly add in more drama than normal if they don't have to? Instead of training adults to be adults, expecting men and women to be respectful professionals, it's simply easier for companies to talk and virtue signal.

It's natural, even reasonable, that managers and human resources staff would avoid hiring anyone who seemed like a sexual harassment case waiting to happen. This might not be fair, but humans aren't known for being rational and mature.

Most employers would gravitate to the candidate who presents a lower risk for potential future problems. A male boss wants someone he can promote without being accused of favoring her solely because she is attractive or talk of an affair, no matter how baseless. A female boss doesn't want an employee that creates more work for her. Her job isn't to babysit one employee, making certain the men don't act like dogs and the women keep their claws to themselves. I know this is not the case one hundred percent of the time. There are male bosses who don't automatically sexually harass female employees, and there are female employees who can become genuine friends. It's just that the probability of this sort of thing happening is so much higher for anyone who has had enhancements or cultivated an exotic dancer's look.

For those who think I'm exaggerating, I wish I were. Because I look a certain way—have had breast augmentation and butt implants, have long hair, full lips, and a fit body because I train three hours a day—men objectify me, and women assume I want to sleep with their men. For the record, I don't.

Now, mind you, I have never had a habit of running around in hot pants and hooker heels. I have always dressed conservatively. This means that the total strangers who routinely hurl insults at me at malls, airports, and grocery stores are forming their opinions based on nothing other than I am, in their minds, too attractive. I'm called a slut, whore, trash, and worse, even in front of my husband and kids. Complete strangers feel entitled to abuse me verbally for no reason other than how I look.

For example, when I was first working on this book, I ran up to the grocery store with my husband to pick up food for the weekend.

My hair was slapped in a ponytail, and I had on a t-shirt, yoga pants, Uggs, a puffy coat, and no makeup. Hardly "porn star" costuming there. The entire time I shopped, a group of teenage girls and boys followed, pointing at me while calling me the standard "slut," "whore," "skank," etc., just loud enough for me to hear. They also said terrible things about me, how I was probably a prostitute, or was trolling the store for a hook-up, how I was totally fake and plastic from behind their hands, all while giggling and not caring at all how their words might actually hurt me. They were having the best time tearing me down. To what end? I have no idea. I continued shopping as if they weren't there. When my husband rounded the aisle and caught them mid-jeer, I had to intervene before things got ugly. He was livid, but I told him to just let it go.

I was used to it.

But should anyone be used to this?

If I can't even go shop for food without facing a gauntlet of mean girls and creeps, then what are the odds that an exotic dancer is going to stand a chance working any sort of professional job unless she's willing to sacrifice being attractive? Why should she be required to be plain or even dowdy to be treated with dignity or respect? She shouldn't. If my personal anecdote above demonstrates anything, it's that clothing choice alone isn't enough to protect her from unfair judgement. In my case, since dressing like a regular mom and being married almost twenty years isn't enough to stop complete strangers from calling me a "whore," I suppose I could cut off my hair, gain fifty pounds, and take up chain-smoking and tanning beds so others won't feel threatened and act like jerks.

Or not.

The same can be said for the exotic dancer. There comes a point a wardrobe change won't be enough. If she permanently reverses everything that makes her 'alluring,' she's risking not making it on the outside and having no way of returning to the profession she knows will pay her bills.

That's a hell of a gamble. And why should she be asked to make it? What right do we as a society have to judge her by her appearance? But judge we do. It isn't right, but it is reality.

The dancer's appearance not only can cage her into the stripping profession, but it also isolates her in a world that is competitive to the point of being merciless. The world of stripping is competitive to the point of being cutthroat. House moms—usually older women staffed to run the show behind the scenes—rule the dressing rooms for good reasons.

House moms are there to make sure a performer's makeup and costume are taken care of, and that she is ready to go on stage. Some even sell costumes to the dancers. Yet, house moms are there namely to keep the dancers from clawing each other's eyes out.

Of course, there are always exceptions, and I'm not saying this is true in all cases, but dancers can be highly territorial, fierce when it comes to getting a leg up, and ruthless when handing out retribution for a real or perceived slight.

Some are not above stealing another dancer's tips, destroying her makeup, shredding her costumes, or trashing her personal belongings, which is why the house mom's role as a behind-the-scenes peacekeeper is extremely important.

A lot of girls who are working as strippers started out pretty rough and hardened to begin with, and they're not to be crossed. Simple math tells us that at any given club, there are obviously going to be more dancers than "whales," or high-end clients. This means the girls will do whatever they can to catch, keep, or even steal those big-fish patrons.

When I was a dancer, I had clients who would show up and just write me large checks. Those were the guys every girl wanted, the customer willing to pay you enough money to excuse you from dancing, keep you off the stage and off your feet for the whole night while buying you drinks.

This is one of many reasons why stripping is very literally survival of the fittest. There really is no camaraderie in a workplace where if you let down your guard for a moment, another dancer could slip in and steal your meal ticket. Everyone is working to locate that Prince

Charming in the audience with the cash to keep you at his table the entire night, all the while knowing there are a thousand frogs to every prince.

Working as an exotic dancer means long hours wearing nothing more than a thong, heels, makeup and a smile. You are constantly selling drinks and hustling for tips and upgraded services like private lap dances. It is long hours dealing with drunks, college frat packs, bawdy bachelor parties, sleazy businessmen, and borderline psychos who might lurk in the audience.

A dancer is always vulnerable to fans who turn into stalkers. It might be the super fan who is paying her the big money to have her at his table for the night who crosses over to wanting more. He doesn't just want to have her. He doesn't want anyone else to have her. Granted, most of these possessive show-off type clients are gold for a dancer, but some can be like having a pet tiger and should be handled with a large helping of caution.

Then there is the polar opposite of the show-off type. He's the broke guy who's jealous of the big shot who can afford to take the prettiest girl—the girl he wants—and keep her all to himself for the whole night. This guy could be the sort who would eventually work up the nerve to take by force what he can't pay to get in the club. He is the loose cannon who will wait and follow that girl into a parking lot or worse, home where her children are sleeping.

This isn't fear mongering on my part. I have seen it happen, had it happen to me, and it's commonly acknowledged as one of the many dangers that just comes with the job.

When I worked as a dancer, we rarely left right after closing and instead, hung around long after to give plenty of time for the members of the audience to clear the parking lot. Even then, the bouncers escorted each of us to our cars as an additional precaution. On top of that, I frequently took different routes home, often doubling back and winding around in very inconvenient paths to wherever I lived on the off chance anyone might be trying to follow. I had already endured a stressful day balancing being seductive and playful with being smart and hyper-vigilant, only to leave exhausted and having to remain on red alert until I was home behind a locked door with the alarm set.

And the next day, I'd do it all over again.

They say insanity is doing the same thing over and over but expecting a different outcome. Like the other areas of adult entertainment, stress, shame, and the basic demands of the job commonly lead to high rates of addiction. Many dancers have to be drunk, high, or stoned simply to cope with who they are and the job they do. That and pushing drink sales is yet another requirement, since each stripper can only be on stage for brief periods of time.

Clubs make most of their money from alcohol sales. The more drinks a dancer sells, the more everybody wins. The guy is buzzed and ostensibly enjoying himself while tipping better. Management is happy because of the nice profit margin on booze sales. A dancer might be invited to sit down with her client while he drinks. She can get off her feet, possibly sell other services like private dances, and her own buzz makes her work more bearable.

Alcohol can numb negative emotions and remove inhibitions. Drinking on the job makes a dancer seem more social. What client wants to drink alone? A strong buzz and lowered inhibitions help her slip into the seductress role more convincingly so she can coax out that extra cash. But there can be a high price to pay. I have seen women get so drunk they fall off stage, some ending up badly injured with broken arms or legs. The habit of tossing back drink after drink, day after day, increases the odds she will end up battling alcoholism.

Also keep in mind that stripping is a highly competitive profession and if a dancer lets herself go, drinks too much, does too many drugs, and fails to remain vigilant, this can easily lead to a demotion or even a pink slip.

Then, we can't ignore the simple truth that a woman who is under the influence is dramatically increasing her risk of being raped or worse.

Mind dulled, she fails to see red flags or isn't as cautious. For instance, instead of keeping an eye on her drink or who's behind her, she becomes overconfident or, conversely, too relaxed. This opens the window of opportunity for a predator to drug her then take advantage. I know because this happened to me.

Then there are the more banal, but still highly stressful, problems. A dancer is beholden to shifts, her days tied to the club and whatever events or needs they might have, or if someone else calls in sick, fails to show, or gets canned. The money isn't entirely predictable because it mostly depends on how many patrons happen to darken the doors of the establishment on any given day. Income is dictated by how much a girl makes in tips or how many customers she can convince to pay for extras. She could work all week and make barely enough to cover the gas it took to drive to and from work, only to turn around and earn more in one night than she did the entire month. It's all a high-stakes gamble at the dog track, only betting on a different breed.

Any money the dancer makes, of course, isn't all hers to keep. The club and other support staff receive a cut because, without the club, the bouncers, waitstaff, and house mom, the dancer couldn't do her job.

Her cage can also be her community, as in the area she calls *home*. She is working either in the locality where she lives or at least close enough to commute. Every time she sets a stiletto on stage, she is risking that someone in the audience will recognize her. Social media is all about the six degrees of separation, and, with facial recognition software, tagging, and mutual friends, this is a constant roll of the dice that no one puts two and two together and blows her alternate identity either out of spite, such as an angry ex getting revenge, or simple ignorance, like a slip of the tongue at the company picnic in earshot of the wives.

Women have always been judged far more harshly than men, for the part they play in the world of adult entertainment. If a dancer has a son, then her son's little league coach wouldn't have to do nearly as much explaining about how he happened to be in a topless bar as she would have to do as to why she happened to be working there.

Strippers also find it all but impossible to date, and when they do date, their partners are frequently abusive, controlling, and jealous.

When you are a stripper, your self-image can't help but end up cracked, warping your perception of what's caring and protective versus controlling and abusive.

Even if, somehow, a girl was able to keep her head high, what kind of man is going to be in a long-term relationship with a stripper? The moment a man finds out what she does for a living, she's diminished in some way. Why? Who knows? Maybe this is because our culture has a Victorian hangover about the value of virginity. We feel the need to categorize women, slot them into "saints" or "sluts." Maybe our culture believes the "damaged woman" is also somehow also a "morally irredeemable woman." I don't have the answers to this, but I do know we need to be asking the questions.

What I can say from personal experience is that most "good guys" wouldn't want to bring a stripper home to mom, thus leaving a pool of male dating candidates no "good girl" would go near.

But strippers are human. We get lonely and need companionship and a sense of safety. Deep down, many accept that beggars can't be choosers and resign themselves to tolerating the intolerable. It's all so when they lock that door at night, they are not alone. They would prefer to be caged with the beast they know than risk facing off the monsters they don't.

Just like any other commission-based salesperson, a dancer can have good days and bad days. Those bad days when the club is empty or clients skimp on tips could mean working extra shifts or events to make up any shortfall.

She could have clients offer hundreds or even thousands of dollars for her to service them outside of the club—what we call "prostitution-lite." At this point, a dancer might venture into intermittent escort work to supplement her income. Most escort services now advertise and operate online, so her picture, vitals and the name she performs under are all listed so potential clients can see who they want to make a date with, but we will address this area of adult entertainment in greater detail in a moment.

When it comes to exotic dancing, I cannot stress this enough: time is continually shrinking her cage. No one remains young, fit, and beautiful forever. Stress and addiction can put a lot of years on a woman almost overnight. There will always be fresher faces and fitter bodies entering the ring as her competition.

As the dancer ages, she will soon find that there is a downward career path for most of those who remain in this business. Maybe she will see it coming and simply have no idea how to do anything else. Or, if she is battling addiction, time passes quickly, and it seems to vanish when she is constantly high, drunk, or stoned. Like many addicts, she believes she can start over, squeeze out a little more time, maybe even find a client who will be her white knight. A dancer might begin at a high-end gentlemen's club, but someone newer and younger will replace her just as she replaced the woman before her. It's inevitable.

In spite of boob jobs, butt implants, Botox, and fillers, if she remains in this business, she will stumble down the ladder, rung by rung, from Night Girl to Day Girl, and then to clubs of lessening prestige until she can only find work at establishments where the clientele can't afford to make it rain crisp hundred-dollar bills all night.

She might have begun in a place where clients flashed company credit cards and racked up thousands in "entertainment" and "business" expenses. But if she gets stuck in stripping long enough? The end of the road is lined with clubs where no one in the audience has an expense account.

Changing One Cage for Another

As an exotic dancer either makes less money because of her age, requires more money to feed an addiction, or has to support a toxic partner or family, she might eventually get desperate enough that she will have little choice but to step out of the stripper cage and into the escort cage, and even possibly the porn cage, in order to augment her income.

First, we will talk about escort work. Some exotic dancers might have had a handful of choice clients they serviced regularly for a steady stream of additional income. But she is an escort, not a wife, and is therefore easily replaced. A high-paying regular can grow bored and spot that fresh new face he would rather pay to make house calls. She is now lost that flow of cash that allowed her to keep dancing as her primary occupation.

There will come a point where choice will be removed. Escort work, once done on the side, becomes an added full-time necessity for any woman who has failed to find another escape. Not only that, but for a woman to gain access to regular clientele and have any shred of safety, the dancer-turned-escort will have to partner with an agent or agency, which I could argue are basically nicer terms for pimp. This is where many dancers trade one cage for another, leaving stripping for escort work.

The Escort Cage

Escorting is a strange arena within adult entertainment that is extremely diverse. This business runs the gamut from girls who hold court with the upper echelons of society to escorts who are only a few steps above streetwalkers and truck stop hookers.

The exotic dancer who has exhausted her marketability on stage will frequently shift to the latter sort of escorting. Sometimes boyfriends act as their pimp, driver, and pseudo-bodyguard. Or they might get work through a home-run operation that pays for the ads, fields the calls, then takes a percentage. She might freelance, placing her own ads online, then rely on a partner to act as driver and bodyguard.

Not everyone ends up in escorting or escorting in the same way, and, like other areas of adult entertainment, escort work can offer plenty of advantages. High-end escorts with a wealthy and powerful client base have the potential to earn not only thousands of dollars an hour but could also enjoy other benefits such as expensive gifts, luxurious travel, and special favors similar to the ones I listed earlier for favorite dancers.

Please keep in mind that there does exist that rare exception of escorts who, like dancers, venture into some other area of adult entertainment, harness the high pay and flexible schedule, parlaying these short-term benefits into long-term gain: a degree, profession, business, or investment portfolio. But all too often, time passes, and the escort, no matter how she ended up an escort, realizes she has missed her window for escape and finds herself caged.

Also, you will soon see that even the most careful and business savvy can never be certain they have truly escaped the Trap. Anyone who does any work in adult entertainment, especially in the modern age, is never fully free.

Escorts might not provide any sexual services, though many do. This is a very gray area, even in the law. Depending on what state, city, or county an escort operates in will impact what is considered completely legal versus a chargeable offense. I'm hesitant to lump all escort work in with prostitution, because the words *escort* and *prostitute* aren't neatly interchangeable. All this aside, though, the same patterns appear in escorting as in other areas of adult entertainment.

Some women transition to being an escort from other areas like webcamming or dancing. Others might go directly into escort work because of the discreet nature of the business. Unlike exotic dancing, it's far simpler to remain anonymous and operate under the radar when working one-on-one with clients who also prioritize discretion and privacy. Since pay can average anywhere from a couple hundred an hour to a couple thousand or even more, escorts can earn more in a few hours than they could earn in a week or even a month at a regular job. Escort work is appealing for women attending college, since they can maneuver work around their student schedule and have time to make their studies a priority.

Yes, as an escort, the pay can be mind-bogglingly good, but like with exotic dancing, an escort is racing against time. She isn't going to remain young and in demand forever. She might begin by refusing to offer or accept performing any illegal service, but age and desperation wear away at her boundaries until they collapse. She doesn't get as many calls, or the clients demand more because they sense she is just desperate enough to agree. The quality of the clientele steadily declines as the rich and powerful begin wanting to try out the newer, fresher "girls."

In fact, it was the rush to find and recruit a steady new stable of escorts in order to attract and grow the list of powerful and wealthy clientele that gave the notorious Hollywood Madam, Heidi Fleiss, her start. When Fleiss was twenty-two, she started managing Madam Alex's girls in the greater Los Angeles area. She also worked as a prostitute so she could learn every aspect of the business.[1]

At the time, Madam Alex had a problem. The women in her employ were aging and looking to retire, so the madam tasked Fleiss with recruiting a new group of young and attractive women to revitalize her struggling business. In 1990, Heidi Fleiss cut ties with Madam Alex to launch her own agency, earning a million dollars in her first four months of operation.[2]

The young women in Fleiss' employ catered to high-ranking politicians, famous actors, professional athletes, judges, and other members of society's elite. Fleiss' good fortune, however, didn't last long. In 1993, she was charged with multiple counts of pandering, and, in 1994, the Feds took Fleiss and her agency down for good and sent her to prison—a very literal cage.[3]

The likes of Heidi Fleiss, however, are rare examples. There are certainly elite agencies who continue to provide services to the rich, famous, influential, and high-profile customers. The higher end escorts don't need to work long hours and can operate largely unnoticed, catering to a cadre of clients who guard their privacy because they appreciate that they, too, are taking a great personal risk by having essentially a paid mistress. Therefore, it's in these types of client's interests to treat their escorts well. Any bad behavior on the client's part could place them in the crosshairs of a devastating, potentially career-ending scandal.

As with all other areas of adult entertainment, there are similar benefits, but they don't come without potentially exacting a hard and heavy price. Even a woman as powerful as Heidi Fleiss was still sentenced to seven years in prison. Many escorts are working in cities where prostitution is illegal. Escorting, by and large, walks the thin tightrope between legal and illegal, so there's always the risk of ending up on the wrong side of the law.

Even escorting services that don't offer actual sex can come under fire, especially during election years when mayors or sheriffs want to project the image of being tough on crime. Thus, an escort who might only offer a private version of what would be completely legal in a strip club—a private strip-tease, for instance—could be rounded up in a vice sting, swept up in a dragnet with actual prostitutes.

Escorts, like the dancers and the webcammers we have already addressed, can also become accustomed to a certain level of income and lifestyle. Money becomes harder to make without sadder compromises and steadily vanishing standards.

Just like the exotic dancer, many escorts suffer the same psychological and emotional trauma, stress of leading a double life, and other hurdles that make leaving this kind of work so difficult, such as the gap in work history, lack of professional training and experience, tell-tale plastic surgery enhancements.

While escorts also deal with all the same sorts of locks as other areas of the sex industry: financial, damaged self-esteem, isolation/lack of healthy support system, and addiction, they might, ironically, run into a wholly unique lock.

They know too much about very important people.

Playing courtesan to those who have a lot of power can make finding professional work challenging. Few customers are eager to hire, or run in the same circles, with a woman who knows all their secrets. Thus, an escort could potentially be directly or indirectly blackballed. For instance, our escort might have paid for her law degree honestly enough, and she might even make an excellent junior attorney. But judges and other lawyers aren't above basic human self-preservation and are wont to prioritize their own futures first. This means distancing themselves, and colleagues, from the escort as if she were radioactive.

The escort cage can be a hard and dangerous business, especially for those who have had to make that tough choice to shift from one form of adult entertainment like stripping or webcamming to essentially a more discreet version of prostitution. First of all, the body takes an entirely new form of abuse. Multiple clients might mean multiple sex partners all in the same day which means sustained and repeated physical trauma. Infections and even sexually transmitted diseases (STDs) are also ever-present threats.

This is all because, obviously, escorts are working in direct contact with clients as opposed to performing remotely via webcamming or on a stage in a strip club that forbids or strictly limits any kind of physical interaction. Clubs also have large bodyguards present to enforce house rules, and to walk the performers to their cars at the end of the shift and guard their safety.

Escorts, on the other hand, have very little protection in their work. Agents and agencies can do some preliminary vetting and can create a client list of "safe" contacts. The level of vetting, obviously, varies from agency to agency. Some might require a client to present valid ID and keep track of anyone who fails to follow the rules. For instance, they would blacklist any client who got too rough, too drunk, too stoned or high, or who invited buddies to join when the agreed appointment was supposed to be a one-on-one session. Access to a list of "safe" customers is a major reason a lot of escorts pair up with an agent or agency. Freelance escorting, by contrast, is extremely dangerous.

Escorts, especially those who freelance, can bring a driver/bodyguard along for protection. Even with safeguards, though, she will largely have to rely on her wits. After all, the bodyguard can only go as far as the door and then the escort is on her own. Once she's alone with the client, it's up to the escort and her intuitive abilities in spotting flags—big, small, and red. A young, inexperienced escort or one struggling with an addiction, can miss major cues when something is seriously amiss and potentially dangerous or even deadly.

Despite precautions, escorts can be robbed or even violently assaulted. Since prostitutes and escorts engage in high-risk behavior as part of their job, they have historically been among the group that human predators routinely target because those who abuse them know these women will always be low on law enforcement's priority list. It's only very recently that escorts could even report being raped to law enforcement. What's sad is the landmark case that finally recognized prostitutes could be raped came at a terrible cost, and only after someone deemed "a proper rape victim" was brutalized.

According to Laura Italiano's April 16, 2010, article in the *New York Post*, "Prostitute Finally Gets Justice in Rape,":

> *When a Manhattan prostitute cried rape in 2006, cops at first did not believe her, leaving the rapist free to rape a second woman two years later....Her attacker, Kevin Rios, was convicted of raping and robbing the terrified woman during a knifepoint attack during a trick-turned-nightmare in a West Side parking lot. "You're a hooker — I can kill you and no one would even care," the pretty victim had testified that Rios, 23 of Spanish Harlem, taunted her while he and a never-captured accomplice raped her in her minivan. Only when Rios was linked to the 2008 knifepoint rape of a Harlem babysitter—by DNA from the prostitute's crime scene—did cops track her down and prosecute, according to law enforcement sources.* [4]

Despite this sort of legal progress, reality has yet to catch up. Even though sex workers now have the right to report rape and be taken seriously, shame will keep many victims silent.

Sometimes, these workers attract the worst of all predators: men who desire to hurt, maim, and kill women.

Granted, this is the direst end of what can happen in this business, but it bears mentioning since whenever there is a serial killer on the hunt, sex workers are usually the most common targets, even today.

One prime example is The Craigslist Killer, also known as the Long Island Serial Killer (LISK), who is believed to have murdered sixteen to twenty people over the course of twenty years.[5] Though plenty of theories abound, LISK's true identity is still unknown. This said, prostitutes and escorts account for the majority of LISK's victims.[6]

One could also add in Ed Kemper, Willie Pickton, the Butcher

Baker of Alaska, the Green River Killer and many other serial killers, all of whom targeted prostitutes and got away with it for so long because law enforcement was so dismissive of the victims. In fact, the only reason Ed Kemper was apprehended was because he called and turned himself in. Before that infamous phone call, Kemper wasn't remotely considered a potential suspect.

Setting aside all the worst-case-scenarios, my goal here is to pull back the veil and expose the reality for performers in the adult industry. Yes, some escape temporarily, but the Trap is very real, and the stakes can be literally life or death.

The Porn Cage

As I hope you see, many of the careers in adult entertainment have a lot of crossovers. It isn't unusual for models to become strippers to become escorts, webcammers to turn to escorting, or escorts to add in webcamming. The only form of adult entertainment that doesn't automatically involve a digital presence is the exotic dancer. Webcammers, escorts, and anything involving online pictures, platforms, or video uploads are parts of the internet, the native soil where the Trap thrives.

Obviously, not every entertainer is going to end up working in porn movies, or what I'll just refer to as *porn* from here. With the digital age, most of the major players such as *Playboy*, *Penthouse*, *Hustler* and other print giants are no longer relevant. Some limp along in digital but have found monetization near impossible when competing with new leviathans such as Pornhub and RedTube. Most of the print pornographers have gone bankrupt and faded away, remembered only as relics of the twentieth century. The digital medium and business model lends itself more to webcamming or video. Why pay to stare at static pictures of naked women when one can log onto any number of sites and watch every erotic scenario the mind can fathom?

All roads can potentially lead to porn; all cages can potentially become the porn cage. With the right triggers, almost anyone can end up trapped in porn. This area of adult entertainment can be one of the most damaging in every aspect, which we'll go into in a moment.

Though strippers have historically been the least likely group to turn to porn, it does happen for any number of reasons. In my case, the trauma from being drugged and raped became a major factor.

A stripper who has aged out of dancing and getting the choicest escort clients could also see porn as a reasonable option. She is all but unemployable outside of adult entertainment anyway and has grown hardened to a life of exploitation. Additionally, she already possesses the basic ingredients required for working in porn:

- she is psychologically and emotionally damaged;
- she has no support system or a parasitic one;
- she probably has any number of telltale augmentations like massive breast implants she now can't afford to have removed;
- she's financially desperate; and
- she has a resume that either lacks many mainstream or office/professional skills, or it has large unexplained gaps of time when she was working in the adult entertainment industry.

Another factor that could play into a dancer's decision to move into porn is simple geography. Consider the area of the country a stripper happens to be working in. An exotic dancer in Rusty Muffler, Oklahoma simply isn't going to bring home the same money as a girl in New York City, Dallas, or Las Vegas.

Moving for work is generally seen as socially acceptable but moving for socially unacceptable work is generally a losing proposition. It's not just about the usual logistical headaches and packing hassles everyone—even strippers—have to deal with when pulling up stakes. Moving means leaving behind friends, family, even a club where at least you know the score. Beyond all that, think of trying to argue that you should keep primary custody of the kids even though you are moving out-of-state for a better job as a stripper.

Even if the dancer does make the move, she has no guarantee the gamble will pay off. Maybe she is considered Night Girl material in a small town, but she might not even be a Day Girl contender in bigger, more crowded, more sophisticated markets. That, and no Night Girl escapes the passing months and years that will one day demote all Night Girls to Day Girls, no matter where she is.

It is therefore not surprising that our small-town dancer might find that getting into making porn is far more doable than scoring a prime performance slot at the finest gentlemen's clubs. So long as an entertainer is somewhat attractive or has something to offer for a niche and willing to do the work, porn provides a path to much higher pay.

Webcammers might not have to deal with geography, demotions, or learning how to sashay while balancing a tray full of drinks and wearing only a thong and plexiglass platforms. But, as I said earlier, webcamming is extremely competitive, and the transition from the webcamming cage to the porn cage can happen without the performer's consent or knowledge. Even if a woman chooses to keep webcamming, working twelve to eighteen hours a day six days a week isn't sustainable long-term. If so? What are her options?

If she knows her private sessions are already out there, and someone else is making money, then she has already traded cages. The only difference is if she doesn't actively do porn, the only one making money is the company that sold her out.

Performers see that they have a problem and the only solution that builds on what they have already been doing instead of forcing them to start over is to move from amateur to professional. To continue webcamming and make a decent living, she will have to work smarter, not harder. This means building her name, brand, and fan base. In the beginning, she might have never imagined she would even consider doing porn films. But after becoming desensitized through her own work, she comes to have a different perspective about porn.

From a business and money-making perspective, graduating from private entertainment to public porn star can simply make a bizarre kind of sense to those in survival mode. Porn films are distributed to a wider audience, and that exposure brings a following right to her on a silver platter. She can increase her following exponentially with every film, as opposed to struggling to win over clients one at a time and exhausting herself with webcamming just to convert a single client into a loyal fan.

Filming a professional porn movie usually takes a day, the work lasting typically from 8:00 a.m. to 6:00 p.m. If it's a huge set, requiring multiple scenes, the day can go from 8:00 a.m. to 11:00 p.m. The performer now has a bit of breathing space where she can cut her webcamming hours back to a more sensible workday. Webcamming to working in porn films is a much more organic path due to the nature of the medium. This has not been the case traditionally for stripping and escort work.

Up until the end of 2019, the adult industry had a general sort of pecking order, and most strippers have zero respect for anyone making porn films. Exotic dancers, as a general rule, rarely made the leap to porn unless some outside crisis forced their hand. Then came COVID-19 and the tsunami of closures and foreclosures.

The escort industry has been dealing with similar hardships. Agencies and even pimps have been desperate to get work for their "girls." Any kind of work. When pimps are starving, that is when you know things are really, *really* bad.

Unemployed strippers and escorts have been joining the online gold rush as well, thereby flooding the webcamming arena with even more amateurs.

Every person has his or her own unique motivation for transitioning into the toughest area of all adult entertainment: porn. The porn experience is different for every performer and before I take you on a tour through this particular prison, I'd like to first share how I stumbled from the stripper cage into the porn cage.

Everyone has a unique story, a path that is theirs alone. In my case, being raped changed everything. It was my personal extinction event, a trauma powerful enough to erase who I had always been, rendering me blank, raw and empty.

As a grown woman, I take responsibility for the choices I have made. No one forced me into the world of adult videos. Yet, at the same time, I had suffered a serious trauma that I had no concept of how to handle coupled with nowhere to turn and no resources to help me process what had happened to me in a healthy way. I felt I was to blame, that I'd brought it on myself. How could someone who took off her clothes for money rightfully call herself a victim? I had been just asking for it, hadn't I?

It took me many years to fully grasp how much that first terrible night affected me, the events it set in motion. That gaping psychic wound tore down all my defenses, and brokenness skewed my ability to make decisions.

Reeling and stunned, I was more exposed than ever before. It made me careless and self-destructive to the point that I ended up being drugged and raped a second time shortly after that first attack. This, of course, only unraveled me further.

While in this shattered state, I made what appeared at the time to be short-term choices. I never dreamed they would come with life-time repercussions. I believed I would one day find a way to get free. This isn't to make any excuses. It's simply my story, and the only story I have any authority to tell. In my case, I could not see beyond the moment. I no longer cared about tomorrow because the future no longer existed.

Since I was reeling from the attacks, my self-esteem shattered, when the offer to do porn came my way, I accepted. In my mind, I was disposable and had no value other than being used as some object. If that was the case, then why not accept higher pay?

When you are part of the trash heap, does the layer of the pile really matter?

I was empty inside, hollowed out and going through the motions. Existing, not living. Any goals or dreams or aspirations I might have had vanished. Money was all that mattered, because making it was all I was good for anyway. I was so messed up from anguish and shame that, for me, porn star was the next logical business step from stripper and Night Girl.

I didn't fully appreciate that I'd begun dying inside when my first husband betrayed me before I ever set a heel on stage. Then, to mentally endure the indignities many exotic dancers face, I had to let even more pieces of "me" fall away to remain somewhat sane. Losing myself had been a long, slow, and steady process for years. All that first rape did was yank the cord and finally unplug me as a human being.

I ceased to be a person and became a sort of automaton, filled with cogs and wheels instead of blood and bone. I was trapped in a spin, and this was the one way I believed I could regain some control. Porn meant working when I wanted and only performing in films of my choosing for far more money. I share this with you because what goes on in the porn cage might seem too awful, too bizarre or horrible to believe. It might even be harder to grasp why anyone would enter this world, let alone remain.

Much of our journey, thus far, has been to educate you about the reality of sex work behind the fiction of adult entertainment the Trap wants you to believe. Hopefully, I've also given sound reasons to empathize with the performers. How they end up in sex work, why they do it and why they remain.

The porn cage, being the most extreme of all scenarios, could possibly be the hardest for a regular person to remain open-minded. Maybe it's easier to grasp how a girl or guy might get into filming porn, but far more challenging to accept how or why anyone would stay. How could they accept this world, the mistreatment and victimization?

Those are thorny questions with no simple answers.

I don't share my experience to be melodramatic or for pity. In fact, out of everything in this book, these intimate details are by far the hardest to part with. I have lived most of my life closed and locked, these memories, feelings, and experiences buried deep.

It's terrifying to open up at all, but I'm telling what happened to me because I'm not alone. There are others who have been similarly blindsided and exploited. At their lowest point, their moment of greatest need, they will reach out, but whose hand will be there to help?

Because if our culture continues to heap even more shame onto those who are the most desperate, then young women and men will continue to fall into the Trap. It's the only place that accepts the broken because it feeds on the violated and profits from pain.

Thus far, we have toured every major area of adult entertainment and only lightly touched on what goes on within the professional adult film industry. You now know how a woman and/or man might end up here, but what then?

As to why any performer continues with sex work, it goes far beyond money, emotional damage, or trauma. There is a difference between being trapped and the Trap. One is a feeling, the other is a digital age monster more insidious than most can fathom, but please be patient. We will talk about the invisible layers of the Trap, the most powerful, in the next chapter because this aspect of the Trap impacts porn actors more than any other area of sex work.

Pulling Back the Curtain

First of all, remember that everything in porn is an illusion. It is entertainment, a performance, and not reality. I have mentioned some of this as we have gone along. This section hopefully will remove any magic from porn because there is nothing magical about it.

Just like world-famous illusionists don't really make people, cars, or planes really disappear, wild horny people aren't having mind-blowing sex on set all day every day. Performers don't enjoy being ravaged by multiple partners. They aren't ecstatic about being gang banged, beaten, tied up, chained, choked, humiliated, or sexually violated with mechanical contraptions.

There are no roving bands of oversexed cougars—any woman over the ripe old age of twenty-five or so—salivating over teenage boys or young men. There are no hordes of hot older moms lying in wait for just the right moment to pounce on their "stepsons" or their "son's friends" and show them seventy-five ways to get off using common household appliances. There aren't gaggles of nymphomaniac cheerleaders holding slumber parties that spontaneously turn into wild orgies.

Even the amateur porn that has recently become so popular is a ruse. There aren't any hidden cameras catching people unawares having crazy threesomes in the back room of a business. The actors know they're being filmed. There is no gotcha. At least not in any legal films.

These are all storylines. They're fiction crafted to seem like reality.

Just like a magic show, porn is a skillful act designed to fool people into accepting the impossible.

If ordinary people ever knew how magicians pulled off their unbelievable stunts, we would lose all awe, and the magicians would be out of a job. This is why escape artists, illusionists, and magicians closely guard how they do what they do.

Porn is very much the same. Everything the audience sees is a masterfully orchestrated deception. The deception is what makes it fantasy, which is what makes porn thrilling and a very large reason why viewers return to see more and more.

It's also why the more scandalous, taboo, or unbelievable the act, the more people line up to watch.

Answer this: what's more interesting, a card trick or making a 747 airplane vanish? Which trick do you think an audience could laugh off as lame or fake or have a theory as to how the deception might have been performed? Which illusionist would draw larger crowds, the one who makes a coin appear from behind someone's ear, or the one who levitates himself twenty feet up into the air?

This, in part, explains why the more extreme versions of porn attract more sets of eyes, because what's harder to believe? That a woman enjoys sex with a man? Or that a woman really enjoys sex with ten complete strangers while gagged and suspended from chains?

Sex between one man and one woman is commonplace. Twenty years ago, though, sex between two women or two men was truly risqué, our culture has changed enough that even this kind of sex is so common as to be almost trite. In our modern era, audiences don't need to rent a porn movie or look at girlie magazines when they have plenty of nudity and vivid sex scenes streaming on HBO, Netflix, Showtime, etc.

Aside from maybe an initial voyeuristic thrill, any regular sex scenarios aren't what's going to hook the most attention for the simple reason that they are so utterly ordinary. Even HBO series like *True Blood* or *Game of Thrones* serve up of plenty of kink once only available in adult video stores. Though some who watch porn might begin with the comparably ordinary, few will remain there long because it's too hard to resist the allure of the extreme. Humans are wired to seek out novelty and will seek out the increasingly new and strange. We do this in many areas of life.

Who wants to watch a magician pull a bird from his hat when there is the illusionist across the street who promises to make a skyscraper disappear? On the flip side, the guy with the magic hat and card tricks either has to retire or figure out how to levitate a cargo train if he hopes to keep and build the crowds who pay to watch him perform.

The same applies to porn actors. If they fail to keep wowing the crowds, they will starve. But this is precisely what will eventually make the Trap's hold so strong.

An illusionist known for making airplanes vanish can never return to doing simple sleight-of-hand. He has to keep upping the ante, or he will lose his fans to the guy who can keep performing illusions that continue to break the boundaries of the believable.

The same can be said for porn actors. They can't go from starring in films hyping "the largest gang bang ever" down to relatively boring threesomes. There is no going back, only forward and deeper and deeper into the Trap.

I'm going to pull back the curtain over the porn cage and reveal many of their trade secrets. It's time to point out the Trap's doors, strings, and wires and expose these curated fantasies for what they truly are.

A lie.

The Work

First of all, professional porn can be a career that follows a certain path that can keep an actress working longer and in relative safety. For an entertainer to land steady work for the best pay, she will need an agent, but even this is a massive gamble with a lot of unknown variables.

If a performer signs with a professional agent who is determined to protect the entertainer's interests and safety, she will have more say in what films she will do. More importantly, she will have the option of turning down more extreme scenarios that could potentially cause physical damage or even permanent injury.

Sadly, there is a far greater chance of a naive performer with no understanding of the industry landing in the hands of the wrong sorts of agents. In the world of adult entertainment, agents have a tremendous amount of power. One might even say they have all the power.

When a performer signs with an agent, that agent essentially owns her for the duration of the contract, usually two years. Many women have the misfortune of ending up with bad agents who use the public's misguided perception that all acts on video are consensual and then maximize profits by participating in a form of sex trafficking.

Yes, porn and sex trafficking frequently cross paths, and the entertainers are often as blind to it as the audience. For anyone who watches porn, there is an implied understanding that what you are watching was created with the full consent of those on the screen. But what if this is an illusion within an illusion? Worse, what if it was something dark and heinous masquerading as something benign?

This might be a bit of a brain-bender, so let's go back to my magic show analogy.

Dark Magic

Let's say a magician performs the incredible act of sawing a woman in half. His beautiful assistant obediently slips into a long, bedazzled box propped up on legs. Her head sticks out one side of the box and her feet out the other. She flashes her beauty queen smile as the magician dramatically wraps the box in chains so she cannot escape.

Smoke machines, dry ice, colored lights, and dramatic music give the stage an eerie atmosphere. The magician then withdraws a wicked saw and begins to cut through the box. Everything is fine until suddenly the assistant's demeanor changes. She cries out in pain.

Surely this is all part of the act, right?

You and the rest of the audience watch her scream, beg for him to stop, and desperately trying to escape while the grinning magician continues sawing, and the audience just sits by. It all seems so real, the blood leaking from her mouth, the way she shrieks. You would think she was actually being sawed in half! At some point, the assistant goes limp, and her skin even turns noticeably pale and waxy. What an actress. Wow!

The magician sets aside his saw, tips his top hat, then wheels the two halves of the box apart to demonstrate that his lovely assistant has, indeed, been parted in two. Maybe even some blood sprays onto the magician's fine suit, or ropy viscera flop from the box onto the floor. Though disturbing, it isn't anything you haven't seen in some cheap haunted house. It's unsettling, frightening, intriguing but also riveting.

Hearing the crowd's growing disquiet, the magician instructs the audience to remain calm. He wheels a silk screen in front of the bisected assistant. The music rises, and the lights dim. When he pulls the screen away, the box is empty, and there stands his assistant blowing kisses to the crowd. Ta-da! She's safe and sound, and you feel that was the most incredible trick ever.

But what if, when that screen covered the box, a trapdoor opened, and a mechanical platform lowered the box below stage where a team hustled in and removed and disposed of an actual dead body?

The living assistant is, in truth, an entirely different woman made up to look like the original assistant.

The audience cheers, even though they all just witnessed a gruesome murder. Of course, they are unaware they witnessed a murder and would never stand for such a depraved and heinous act if they knew the truth. But the problem is they have no way of discerning what is real and isn't real.

All they know is they observed something incredible and can't wait to see that magician's next show. Maybe they will even recommend it to friends.

Since this magic act is so popular, drawing so many crowds and making so much money, the magician continues to perform. He might even make the show more gruesome as it goes on or increase the number of shows. As long as the audience has no idea that they are watching actual murders, the murder magic show can continue. In fact, the show can expand due to increased profits from more people wanting to come and see the unfathomable for themselves.

Yes, my example might be a bit over the top, but, as we go along, you will see my made-up story isn't as far off-base as one might imagine.

One of the largest problems with porn is that the notion of consent is routinely abused, especially as the audience's demand for violent and extreme content increases.

The "Consent" Trick

Here is another secret you might not know about porn. What the audience is watching might not actually be consensual at all, or it might be partially consensual. For instance, an actress agrees to do a film having sex with two other men. She did not, however, agree to being tied up, beaten, and raped by five men. The thing is that viewers have no way of discerning if what they are watching was ever consensual at all.

This is why the Trap works so hard to dehumanize sex workers. If it can keep feeding the myth that everything happening on screen is totally legitimate, legal, and consensual, then the audience feels less guilty watching. Because the audience has been fooled, the performers also lose agency and the right to say no.

The performers are the magician's assistant chained in the box. In many kinds of films, the more the performers scream, struggle, fight, or beg, the better the act. This might be consensual or not. The audience can't verify which is true, and that's why they rely on porn sites' assertions that they are moderating all content and everything available has been previously vetted as legitimate.

Once the performers are off-set, what happens then? When it comes to sympathy, why would porn actors want sympathy for something they agreed to and were paid to do? Is it even possible to rape a porn star?

The notion that adult entertainers are somehow less human is one of many lies the Trap requires to keep flourishing. Corporations, international media conglomerates, production companies, agents, advertisers and all others who profit from porn take advantage of the public's understanding of consent and bend any ignorance to their advantage. They don't outright lie when lies of omission work just as well, if not better, because blank space and assumptions allow them to deftly maneuver any legal considerations or blowback.

Viewers watch porn in good faith, trusting that those financing and making the films are following certain laws and guidelines. Audiences, generally speaking, believe they are watching a scripted, fake, consensual, wild gang bang film, when they might actually be witnessing an actual gang rape. Then, because they are watching, they are unintentionally supporting, financing, and emboldening a masterfully disguised form of sex trafficking.

I place heavy emphasis on the word unintentionally. Like the audience members in my make-believe murder magic show, most regular people don't know what really goes on behind the scenes in on a porn set. Regular people don't know the truth because those profiting have a vested interest that audiences remain in the dark so they will keep consuming more content.

In fact, this variety of sex trafficking is so cleverly veiled, most

performers are just as blind to the true legal definition and boundaries that define true consent. Many entertainers have no idea they
have been victimized because the industry beats us down so much
that we tend to accept whatever happens without complaint.

To be clear, obviously not all porn falls into the category of sex
trafficking. However, you might be shocked at just how much of what
porn actors endure actually meets the legal burden for sex trafficking,
at least according to how the United States Department of Justice
defines this crime.

According to the U.S. Department of Justice:

> *Human Trafficking is a crime that involves exploiting a person for labor,
> services, or* <u>*commercial sex.*</u> *The Trafficking Victims Protection Act of 2000
> and its subsequent reauthorizations define human trafficking as: a)* <u>*Sex
> trafficking in which a commercial sex act is induced by force, fraud, or
> coercion*</u> *[Emphasis added], or in which the person induced to perform
> such act has not attained 18 years of age...*[7]

The U.S. Department of Justice specifically cites that commercial
sex (sex for the purposes of profit) falls under the definition of
human trafficking if there is any form of exploitation involved. Sex
trafficking expands the definition of commercial sex and how and
when it crosses the legal line.

**Any commercial sex act that is induced by *force*, *fraud*, or *coer-
cion* counts as sex trafficking.**

Again, how many porn actors realize they have actually been
victims of sex trafficking? I would bet very few. I can honestly say that
until I started doing research for this book, I didn't even understand
that I myself had been a victim of sex trafficking on numerous
occasions.

Why would I think I had? As a society, we have come to collectively think of sex trafficking in a very different way. We envision
small children, kidnappings, and nefarious underground crime
syndicates. Lurid tales of dark web intrigues and online auctions
captivate imagination and monopolize attention. The Trap thrives if

it can keep people distracted with distortions because this serves its agenda. If even professional porn actors don't realize they are being preyed upon by those who twist the concept of consent, why would anyone else?

The misapplication of consent is rampant in porn.

For instance, an actress might believe she has agreed to a film where she is to have sex with one guy, only to fly out to Los Angeles and find it's a whole other ballgame. It is not uncommon for producers, directors, and/or agents to pull bait-and-switches. Only once the actress is on set does she realize the film is actually with three or four men, not the original single partner. Or worse, the script could be a violent sadism & masochism (S&M) scenario where she is tied down and brutalized.

This is fraud. The producers, directors, and agent all knew what the film really entailed, and yet they knowingly and willfully misrepresented about what the actress was agreeing to.

If she says no and tries to back out, she risks being branded as "difficult" and blackballed. Agents frequently threaten to weaponize a performer's contract if she fails to comply. If she doesn't do what she is told even though she never agreed to it in the first place, that agent won't book her for any future work for the remainder of her contract. This means no film work for the next two years. Agents have even gone so far as to threaten to sue performers for breach of contract.

Producers, directors, and even members of the crew have been known to demand sexual favors from a performer. If she refuses, she won't get paid and again risks ending up blacklisted.

Sounds a lot like **exploitation, force** and **coercion** to me.

I have managed to have a longer career than most porn actresses, but that isn't to say I have not suffered through the stuff of nightmares. One time, my agent signed me to do a film described to me as having only "a little light bondage and S&M." Once on location, however, everything went sideways to the point that some of what happened to me is a blur. Time skips around. I recall most of what occurred, but to this day, the exact order of what was done to me remains unclear.

Warning: this next bit includes descriptions of non-consensual sex, non-consensual sadomasochism, suicidal ideation, and bodily damage resulting from extreme sex acts.

I remember arriving, rehearsing my lines while getting into makeup and costume, then the crew tied me up with ropes. That wasn't a surprise. I had come prepared for some bondage. It was only after the crew had me tied up that everything went off script and off the rails.

Once I was totally immobilized, the crew used clamps to pin my eyelids open so I couldn't blink. The director was going for a wild-eyed terrified expression, but he didn't need the clamps because I was plenty terrified. The crew covered my face with suction cups, then jammed metal clamps up my nostrils and then fixed similar large alligator clips over my entire body, including my nipples. All of this was extremely painful, and I couldn't make them stop. I must have kept passing out because I'm still missing sections of time from after I was tied up.

There was some point where I was bleeding, probably from a bloody nose. I vaguely remember someone saying they couldn't have blood in the shot and ordering an assistant to clean the blood off the floor. Then, crew members jammed a ball-gag in my mouth, then hoisted me into the back of a dump truck where male actors took over. In the end, the studio got the scenes it wanted...fear, shock, and brutality.

By the time I finished shooting, I was literally going into shock. I was pale, hyperventilating, and shaking. My whole body was covered in bruises, scrapes, and cuts. My face was badly swollen, and the suction cups left angry round purple whelps that didn't heal for weeks.

On top of the psychological trauma, even though I was sobbing inconsolably, the director ordered me to do an after-interview to convince the audience I was completely fine and had a great time. If I refused, they wouldn't pay me. There was no way I was going to endure all that for no pay, so I went along. After I left, I fell apart. I was hysterical the whole way home and that night came very close to killing myself.

Maybe I'm made of stronger stuff, I don't know. At the time, I had a handful of advantages which afforded me the ability to stand up for myself. First, I was a seasoned performer with years in the adult industry. I possessed knowledge and understanding about the business that a young naive performer likely wouldn't have. I also had a loving husband and family as a support network, all of them ready and willing to fight for me.

My experiences up to that point had also made me an expert at disassociating. I could separate my wrecked self from the hard, no-nonsense, and this-is-not-how-we-will-do-business self for long enough to raise hell. Most importantly, I had already become a brand in the industry, an entertainer with a fan base I could leverage.

I made it through and took my agent to task to make sure nothing like that ever happened again.

But what about the new actress with no emotional support system who isn't a brand, who doesn't wield a strong fan following and has zero leverage? What happens to her? Assuming she doesn't kill herself, she might not know how to push back or even that she can. She might be shattered into so many pieces that she lacks the wherewithal to gather enough of those broken bits together and stand up for herself.

While experienced performers aren't immune from being fooled, generally bad agents and unsavory producers and directors prefer naive and unknown performers since they make the easiest targets A green enough performer is promised one sort of porn only to be rooked into extreme porn. For instance, she ends up agreeing to do double or triple vaginal ,double or triple anal, or some combination of the two.

It doesn't take someone with a medical degree to know this can easily blow out her body almost instantly. What could have been a longer career in regular porn is cut short because these extreme sex acts cause severe anal prolapses, which is when the intestines are literally falling outside of her body because of damage to the anal muscles and colon.

This damage also renders the performer incontinent, unable to control her bladder or bowels. To keep working, she will end up only able to work in extreme films and fetish films. She is the performer who will only get the films with multiple giant penises or foreign objects rammed into every orifice. Because she can't control her bladder or bowels, she will find most of her work is in fetish films for viewers who want to see women take a bowel movement or urinate on themselves or on other actors. If she has a distended bowel (referred to as a *rosebud* in the industry), she will be slated for films that cater to audiences who are aroused watching women play with, lick, or display a horrendously prolapsed colon.

The Acting

There is so much competition for paid work, many performers are afraid to turn down any job because a refusal could put their very livelihood in jeopardy. They have to play the game or risk ending up blackballed. So, no matter what is happening, porn actresses will moan and howl as if they have never had a better experience in their lives, but again, it's an act. They are paid to pretend they are having the time of their lives, and if they aren't convincing enough, they won't get any other film deals.

Meanwhile, porn leads audiences to believe women love anal sex, that they can't get enough of it. What viewers don't know is that performers are paid more for agreeing to engage in anal intercourse. Though obviously I can't speak for every performer, letting down boundaries—like agreeing to anal sex or other more extreme sex acts —is about money, keeping work, and getting more work. That's all. Enjoyment isn't even the smallest part of the equation.

I cannot say this enough, but everything caught on camera is scripted. Actors are on set, surrounded by crew members who manage lighting, sound, filming, makeup, the setting, and costumes. Viewers aren't going to see the crew crammed in on the set, or the adjacent break room where other performers are having a sandwich and texting. They are oblivious to the actress having to sit on ice because she is in pain and bleeding. The viewers have no way to witness the actor slathering more concealer on his privates to cover the herpes sores.

Yes, technically actors are not allowed to work if they have an STD, an outbreak, or infection, but those rules are routinely ignored. It doesn't matter if the performer has a flare up of herpes, a vaginal infection, or a raging case of chlamydia, the show goes on.

An actress might be writhing in ecstasy, only to hear, "Cut!" The director didn't care for the lighting, or thought she should scream louder, or the male actor should be in a different position. Everyone stops until they hear, "Action!" Then, the performers pick up where they left off going through the motions. There is nothing intimate, thrilling, or erotic happening. We, the actors, all might as well be robots. It is a performance, not reality.

The Performers

Humans are attracted to extremes. This is true in the entire film industry. In real life, government spies don't look anything like Hollywood A-list stars. But those who make regular movies know they can't cast ordinary people in these roles. Sexy sells.

Porn is no different. Sure, they're going to cast men with unnaturally large penises and females who've been physically altered to similar extremes with giant breasts or butt implants. Those making and financing the films are also going to keep pushing boundaries every way they can.

The Set

Film sets can range from old, dirty studios crammed with actors and crew to spacious mansions rented out for the day. I once did a film where we (the porn people) were literally entering a location just as the film crew for an episode of *CSI* was leaving.

A girl might be filming in an abandoned hospital or mothballed factory, in a forest, or in someone's kitchen. Like any movie, sets are often chosen to reflect the storyline of a film which could mean anything from a palatial estate to a decommissioned prison.

The only true limitation for professional porn production is the law. Only a handful of states and cities legally permit making porn films, so most of the work is done in three main states, California, Nevada, and Florida, concentrated in cities like Los Angeles, Las Vegas, Reno, and Miami.

In a previous section I mentioned how performers still work even if they are contagious with some STD. When the HIV/AIDS scare hit, the laws changed requiring porn actors to wear condoms. At first the industry complied, but over time, as the panic dwindled, directors decided they didn't care for the optics of condoms. They wanted to show males ejaculating to thrill viewers, and condoms made this cumbersome. Many production companies resolved these issues simply by changing where they made films, for example moving to Nevada which didn't require condoms to be worn.

Though actors and actresses, by and large, continued to keep getting tested regularly for STDs, this didn't really solve the problem. Generally, testing is done every two weeks. The problem is who knows what has happened in the two weeks since the test? For all we knew, the night after an actor was tested, he could have hooked up with someone infected with HIV, gonorrhea, syphilis, or whatever. Sure, his tests show he is clean but is he really?

It's a risk all actors and actresses take every time they make a film. Most porn performers have contracted multiple STDs over the course of their career. We know the odds are, at some point, we will have to be treated for at least the most common STDs, including gonorrhea, chlamydia, herpes, genital warts, etc. Real erotic, right?

This is a good point to mention some other consequences from the COVID-19 pandemic. Since the studios are closed, both professional and amateur entertainers are making films from their own from homes.

Pre-pandemic, the law required performers to be tested every two weeks for all variety of diseases and viruses in order to be medically cleared to work. Yes, these laws were often followed loosely, but there was at least some attempt at a safeguard. Professional studios could only film in certain locations and were required to have permits. Also, there were only professional porn actors in these films. The porn world is a small community, which helped somewhat. Often, we were aware of anyone who had contracted any disease or illness and could steer clear until that performer was safe to work with.

Now, we have a compounded problem in porn. We have everyday people playing porn star who have no idea the kind of rigorous testing they should be getting regularly to make these sorts of videos, especially videos without condoms and with anyone other than their committed, monogamous partner.

Then, many of the pros who have gone indie aren't getting tested because they can't afford it. On top of this, they're also not being tested for COVID-19 before filming, because that's an additional cost they can't cover. This means many highly transmissible and even deadly viruses, including HIV and COVID-19, can start an entirely new outbreak because of a single patient zero in a homemade film.

Tricks of the Trade

Again, porn works much like a magic act. The industry crafts illusions that mess with the audience's mind to make them believe something impossible. **Again, a quick warning: this section covers some graphic content including industry slang, explicit descriptions, and scatology.**

First, we will talk about the promotional pictures, starting with the still photos featuring the *cum shot*, or a man ejaculating. The audience sees an actress with a mouthful of cum. It's all over her face, in her hair, and down her body. First of all, this is a biological impossibility. A man simply can't ejaculate that much fluid. Not to mention the fact that the crew understands the odds of capturing the right cum shot in a photo would be slim-to-none. In a packed production schedule, there is no time for the actor to recover in order to take the picture again.

So, if it isn't real, what exactly is the audience seeing? A prop. The industry uses substances that mimic semen's color and viscosity. I have had to pose while practically gagging on a mouthful of Cetaphil.

Yes, the face cleanser.

I have had Cetaphil in my mouth, dripping down my face, in my hair and all down my body. Fun times. Not. The studio might also use piña colada mixer to create a similar illusion. (Sorry if I just ruined piña coladas for you...at least you still have walks in the rain).

Males can ejaculate for real during the film because their bodies are different. Apply enough friction over time, and a man will orgasm. But, since the studio wants to save the real orgasm for the video, they use trickery for the promotional photos.

There are many other deceptions common in the actual film, itself. Yes, when a woman orgasms, she can "ejaculate" as well, which is referred to as *squirting* in the adult industry. Just as viewers yearn for the cum shot, they also love to see the actress squirt.

This is where basic human physiology, again, gets in the way. First of all, I can promise you that the sex we have on porn set is so rote and fake, so devoid of any intimacy or authentic arousal, that probably most women are not having an orgasm at all, let alone orgasm after orgasm.

Theoretically, even if we were orgasming six times an hour, the female body is not going to produce that much fluid when she climaxes. Then, there is the other inconvenient fact that, unlike a man, we can't be made to have an authentic orgasm simply by applying enough friction.

So, how then can we squirt liberally, on command, and multiple times? Good question. Actresses aren't having an orgasm and ejaculating. They aren't squirting.

They are urinating.

To begin with, squirting is a physiologically involuntary release of a small amount of urine during climax. It's not even something that occurs in all female climaxes. But in order to provide the exaggerated visual porn viewers want, actresses drink absurd amounts of water between scenes, and when cued to climax, we urinate all over the other actor/actors and ourselves. And yes, we moan because we are paid to moan. There might be just the tiniest bit of real pleasure in the sound because by that point, we have had to pee so long it hurts. Our ecstatic cries are really the elated sounds of someone relieving a bladder about to burst.

All kidding aside, you can imagine how grumpy all of us can get between scenes. It's smelly, uncomfortable, unsanitary, and flat out gross.

Even though, as a performer, I've managed to evade the more perverse fetish films, I've seen enough to call foul. Scat films involve using or playing with fecal matter for the purposes of sexual arousal. These films probably are using the same types of deception, or at least I seriously hope they are.

In scat films, the film might, for example, lead the audience to believe that a performer is taking a giant bowel movement into some other performer's mouth, but I'm not wholly convinced. My money is on cake icing, chocolate pudding, or something that only resembles excrement. So, when actresses are rolling around in, licking, or eating "crap," they are probably high on sugar, not the erotic thrill of doing every crazy thing imaginable with human waste.

I want to believe videos of golden showers really are lemonade spouting from hidden tubing, not urine. Scat films? Still hoping for brownie batter squeezed from cleverly hidden pouches, because the alternative—that this is all real—is too much even for me.

All in All...

I imagine that for many of you reading this section was tough. It was tough for me to write, and I've been in the business. But there are so many consequences that come from how the porn industry is constructed, how it operates, and even how it deceives.

The general public often forms an opinion about porn based on emotions, hearsay, and deliberate misinformation, which hardens them to what performers endure. They don't realize the rigors of the job, know how entertainers are exploited, and cannot grasp how little power we have in relation to those who provide us a living. Those who watch porn buy into a lie that the people in the films are having incredible and exotic erotic experiences. The viewers start judging themselves and others using a measuring stick marked with lies big and small. Maybe they feel woefully inadequate because of their bodies, or they believe the partner they once loved is boring or cold. Their once healthy concept of sex steadily slips until fantasy replaces reality and no loving relationship can survive when weighed against an artificial standard.

Men might not understand why their woman isn't having the same orgasms as the women in the films he watches. Is something wrong with him? Or is it his partner? This starts a destructive cycle on the other side of the screen that damages self-esteem, intimacy, and fundamentally alters reality in a way that benefits porn at the expense of in-person relationships.

Yes, I admit it. I stepped into the porn cage of my own volition. What I didn't fully grasp at the time was that I was trading one pain for another pain, one cage for another cage. Porn paid better and demanded less of my time, but it was also a path that led me deeper into the Trap.

I had no full understanding of what kind of trade-off I'd made, the toll it would take, and how I'd unwittingly given myself a life sentence in adult entertainment.

7

THE CHAINS THAT BIND

W hy don't you just leave? Go get a respectable job? You just keep doing porn because you are addicted to sex, greedy, lazy...

For the individual who entered into porn believing she could leave any time she wanted, this is the point where the Trap becomes most obvious because they have decided to leave only to realize all the exits are sealed. Before we go further, I can attest there are plenty of people out there who view porn as a legitimate career and enjoy what they do. It isn't my place to speak for them because, again, I can only speak from my own experiences.

Again, the Trap is only a trap to those wanting to leave, who suddenly realize they can't. Trust me when I tell you that I have tried multiple times to leave porn, and that was before computers had near the power they hold now. Many of us do try to leave, but the public doesn't understand how the deck is stacked against that ever happening, especially in the digital age.

I went back and forth when it came to writing this book because it's difficult not to feel like a hypocrite. Porn has benefited me in many ways. Certainly, many of my fans have been wonderful and support-ive. I have made excellent money, lived a nice lifestyle, and provided well for my family. Being an adult entertainer gave me financial stability and flexibility most regular women never enjoy. Instead of slaving away working two or three jobs, my work schedule allowed me the greatest gift of all...time to be a mom.

Yet, any advantages I have enjoyed have come at a terrible cost. I have spent most of my life feeling like the walking wounded. The nature of porn is to be constantly exposed to danger. Even when you are professional and take every precaution, you still can't always account for everything.

The work has damaged me physically, mentally, and psychologically. I have been badly injured on set and can think of at least three times I almost died filming. Not only do I carry the emotional scars and psychic wounds, but I have also had numerous surgeries on my neck and back. I managed to handle the first surgeries well enough, but as I mentioned earlier, I eventually grew dependent on the pain pills and had to battle my way back from addiction. So, yes, this is not all as glamorous as it might seem.

I'm here simply to tell my truth and make those reading this aware that far too many enter into adult entertainment under duress only to later realize they can't leave. I know this for a fact because here's the thing: if I'd had it my way, I would have long ago left porn to work in a very different profession.

And yes, I wanted to leave this industry. Of course, I did!

But every day I worked in a real job, I risked someone recognizing me. The moment anyone found out who I was, it was game over.

The first time I tried to leave was in 2003 after I earned my nursing degree. I would just get settled into a job when someone would invariably recognize me. It was always only a matter of time until I was being propositioned, cornered, felt up, or fired. So, I went back into adult work to pay the bills. The second time was in 2004 when my husband and I moved our family to Virginia. I couldn't find a job that paid enough, not even in nursing.

In 2005, I tried leaving for a third time by getting my real estate license. Ultimately, I quit for safety reasons. Fans-turned-stalkers would book appointments posing as potential home buyers. Appointments turned into ambushes. I was constantly worried about being followed and actually was followed on a number of occasions.

Finally, I hit a breaking point. I couldn't take the stress of being recognized, stalked, and potentially attacked, so, in 2006, I resumed webcamming to pay the bills, then went back to stripping in Vegas from 2007 to 2008. In 2009, I returned to porn full time. In 2017 I tried a fourth time to leave the industry. A vacation rental company hired me as a manager. I was ecstatic that I could finally have a professional career and a normal life.

But during orientation, one of the hotel's staff members recognized me and complained. My employer immediately called me into a private meeting and fired me on the spot.

I hadn't broken any laws. I was obviously qualified enough to be hired in the first place.

While our culture might not find porn socially acceptable, a lot of it is legal. I've only ever performed with other consenting adults, producing content created for other adults. Yet, one might think I was worse than a sex offender with the way I was treated. Sex offenders, who have broken actual laws, at least can get job placement assistance after serving their sentence.

Why is it illegal to discriminate based on a person's race, gender, sexual orientation, religion, disability, marital status, etc., but it's completely fine to discriminate against a person if they have ever worked a legal job in adult entertainment?

Each and every time I tried to start building a regular career, it was only a matter of time until others exposed me. I had been branded with a Scarlet XXX. What's really frustrating is that frequently the same people who write us off, who spout nonsense like, "Why don't porn stars just leave and get a real job?" These were usually the same type of people who exploited me, outed me, and ultimately demanded I crawl back down into that trap I had the gall to claw my way out of.

What so much of the public fails to understand is that ignorance only makes the Trap stronger, shackling performers and wrapping them in chains from every direction.

For the entertainer, trying to break out of the industry is much like trying to break out of a Super Max prison. There are many doors, many locks, and ruthless guards between that small room and the outside world. Cameras are everywhere.

Escape is more than, "Why don't you just quit and get a real job?" Examples are everywhere, but throughout the rest of this chapter, I will mention cases similar to my own experiences.

Teacher, Teacher

The first case concerns a woman who worked in the adult industry before the digital age. She believed she could make a new life, and she did...until it all fell apart. This is a perfect example of the Trap.

According to a 2017 article in *The Dallas Morning News*, "A sixth-grade teacher at an all-girls academy in Dallas ISD says she was fired after word got out that she was an adult film actress more than 16 years ago."[1]

Resa Woodward, who taught science at an all-girls STEAM Academy, had worked in education for fifteen years and had even earned a master's degree. She admitted to being in porn, but made it clear to her employers that it was not a career of her choosing and was part of her very distant past.[2]

Resa claims that when she was a teenager she was involved in an abusive relationship with a much older man and that he pressured her into working in porn. Once she was able to get free of the situation, she completed college, became a teacher, and continued working in education for most of her adult life.[3]

Despite all she had overcome, all her hard work came crashing down when the district received an anonymous tip publicly revealing Resa's past and that her film name was Robyn Foster.[4]

Again, this same article mentions that, "'The caller was concerned because he/she did not want his/her child exposed to things like this,' according to the report. The tipster felt Woodward was trying to deceive the students and parents."[5]

Wow. What a good citizen.

Exposed to what? A really good teacher with fifteen years of experience and a master's degree who was teaching hard sciences and encouraging girls to get into STEAM? A teacher who no one would have ever known worked in porn without this helpful citizen's tip?

Instead of focusing on Resa's story of redemption and overcoming adversity—escaping a bad relationship, leaving the adult industry, earning advanced education and dedicating herself to a noble career —the district, parents, public and media fixated, instead, on her past. If you google *Resa Woodward*, what you will find, other than an abandoned LinkedIn profile, is page after page, article after article obsessing over her scandal and disgrace. There is hardly a mention regarding what she overcame and what she accomplished.

Resa Woodward's decade and a half serving as an exemplary educator have all been relegated to brief mentions and footnotes. As much as I tried to find out what became of Resa, the internet seems to only care that she was once a porn star who dared to forget her place and try to become something better, or worse, a teacher.

Even though Resa Woodward left before porn went digital, all it took was one anonymous tip to set in motion a chain of events that eventually destroyed her career, her name, and her life. I don't know what has become of Resa, so yes, I am working with conjecture. But, even if she's somehow managed to rebuild some kind of life, imagine how hard that had to be. Her name is and will forever be linked to a past she'd worked hard to escape. She *believed* she was free.

And you know what? Maybe she was in an abusive relationship, and maybe she was pressured into the industry, but why does it matter? Why did any of that matter?

Why did information from an anonymous tip about films this woman made in 2001 matter in 2017? What lesson did this teach to a generation of young girls attending an all-girl school with a mission of female empowerment?

Don't ever make a mistake because you will be hunted down and punished. You can't hide, and you will never EVER be forgotten or forgiven.

I suspect that, even if Resa manages to start over, the precautions she will have to take to remain hidden will be extreme. Just think of the constant fear she has been condemned to. Every day, she never knows if this day will be the day her life implodes all over again. Even if she makes it through the day, she will go to bed wondering if tomorrow will be the day her world is shattered once more.

What frustrates me so much is that often many of the same people who secretly consume adult entertainment from the privacy of home are the same people who will out the porn star trying to escape. How else did this "concerned citizen" know about Resa's past life in porn? What should dismay and frighten everyone is that these individuals have no real problem condemning a teacher who has committed no crime to a life sentence without parole or pardon. Meanwhile, her accusers suffer no consequences or condemnation for destroying another human being's life.

In the modern Information Age, the same computer algorithms that hyperlink performers to clients willing to pay money are the same tools fashioning stronger and tighter *links* into the chains that bind.

Brave New Porn

This isn't 1980. Everyone has a computer. We are almost a cashless society. Privacy no longer exists. We are truly a global economy, all connected digitally via extraordinarily sophisticated technology currently exerting unchecked power and influence.

It might be easy for some reading this to think I sound like some conspiracy theory nut, but when was the last time you applied for a job?

Even a simple application to Walmart is run through a computer filter. Then, let's say someone wants to leave porn and secure a job that requires any kind of resumé. What is the first thing you have to do when applying for a job? Write a cover letter that hits all the keywords and a resume that does the same because software will sift through all those applications and automatically reject any that don't play the keyword game. Companies don't even have to invest in developing this technology themselves. They can simply pay a fee to employment posting aggregators such as Monster and ZipRecruiter who promise to deliver the choicest "hand-picked" candidates right to their inbox.

In the name of improving efficiency and saving time, recruiting software runs almost every job application packet through a formidable gauntlet of advanced filters and search programs powered by self-evolving algorithms. These sorts of searches are meant to winnow through and automatically reject as many applicants as possible.

There is no sense in wasting company time and money interviewing someone who is inappropriate or under-qualified. For instance, say a jewelry store is hiring new salespeople for the holiday season. Anyone with a low credit score, a recent bankruptcy, or who is in massive debt is an automatic "No."

Many software programs harness state-of-the-art software to crawl the web, searching for keywords that might warrant automatic rejection. As systems advance, employers are adding more and more virtual layers between a prospective applicant and that first in-person interview.

But say a performer makes it through the screening process and reaches the point where she is a serious candidate for a job. The next step is often a background check. This used to entail only searching for whether or not the potential candidate had a felony criminal record or maybe running a credit check. Now, many companies either have departments or hire outside security consultants who have the resources to scour the web in search of everything and anything potentially damning. This is largely why so many entertainers who try to leave can only gain access to low-paying, low-skill jobs. Those jobs usually only run a cursory check, at least for now. Any professional positions, however, would automatically be off the table because most entertainers would be unlikely to pass the background check.

We live in a digital fishbowl. Everything we do online is collected and stored forever. Though I will go deeper into this topic later, for now we will keep it simple. Privacy is a myth. What happens in Vegas stays on Google forever.

Hotel Silicon Valley

But, hey, this shouldn't be an issue. After all, nobody in adult entertainment uses their actual name, right? Wrong. Too many people still believe it's possible to keep a legal identity and a made-up porn moniker separate. A potential employer would only use the performer's legal name for a background, not her stage name.

Maybe twenty years ago, but now, the reach of many employers extends into any and all online or social media activity, as well as any and all information that might populate from search engines, social sites, online mailing lists, etc., about an applicant in a search. Currently, many businesses and civilians have access to the same computer algorithms and the same facial recognition software that was once only accessible to agencies like the FBI, CIA, NSA, and INTERPOL. There is no hard delineation between the private/corporate sector and the government/law enforcement sector when it comes to using the internet and social media to extract information.

For instance, when looters and rioters hijacked peaceful protests in Seattle in the summer of 2020 and defaced or even destroyed federal buildings and property, many of the perpetrators believed they would have walked away scot-free. That was until law enforcement agents quickly started rounding them up for federal prosecution, warrants already in hand.

How were so many of these suspects identified clearly enough for law enforcement to not only find them after the fact, but to also have the evidence required to meet the necessary legal burden to obtain arrest warrants? Simply identifying many of the suspects was already quite a feat. Considering many of the suspects had no prior criminal history, this meant that they wouldn't be listed in any law enforcement database.

If the looters weren't already in a criminal database, then how did the government find them? Agents hopped online and accessed the most highly advanced facial recognition software on the planet: social media. Facial recognition software is what makes tagging other people in a photo possible. In cases where investigators couldn't get a clean match to a face, they used filters like geographic location to narrow the pool to likeliest candidates. Then, they scoured those profiles' images for other identifying markers like tattoos, jewelry, or clothing labels until they could make a definitive identification.

Companies running a background check on a potential candidate often do all this and more. This is scary enough, but there is a lot of hidden data that many people don't even realize exists. We also assume we can control our privacy, when that is patently false.

Digital Bondage

The two largest social media sites, Facebook and Instagram, not only have rights to all the images we upload based on the Terms of Service Agreement we all have to click to use the sites, but **they also lay claim to any and all metadata that might be embedded in those images.**

Until recently, social media could only assert rights, ownership, and access to images we posted, as well as any metadata embedded in the image.

Now, if you post using the app from your smartphone—which we all know is way more common and convenient—**Facebook and Instagram have access to all photos on our device, metadata included**, regardless of whether we post them or not.

Granted, you can try to deny access to *all* your photos, but then these sites make uploading any picture so frustrating most users will simply give in, unaware of exactly what they are giving away.

So, exactly what is metadata, and what does it have to do with the adult industry or porn?

Metadata is a fancy word for "data about data." It's encoded information in the very format of a digital file. Most regular people have no idea that the images they post are automatically embedded with metadata. We scroll images on Instagram and Facebook, but those photos are more than just pretty pixels and fancy filters. A digital photo's metadata can reveal where you work, live, vacation, the exact GPS coordinates of where the photo was taken, which can then be plugged into any mapping application. Photos can reveal the exact time and date the photo was taken and even identify what sort of device took the picture.

This is the high price we pay for FREE.

According to the updated December 6, 2019, *Consumer Reports* article by Thomas Germain, "How a Photo's Hidden 'Exif' Data Exposes Your Personal Information,":

> *Details about when, where, and how a photo was taken are captured automatically by smartphones and digital cameras and stored as Exif (Exchangeable Image File Format) data. Information on everything from exposure settings to altitude may be included. And the Exif data travels with the photo—from the camera to your hard drive or a website.* [6]

An entertainer might have a completely separate social media profile under a pseudonym to promote her webcamming side gig that is keeping the lights on after being laid off. She probably doesn't mention where she lives on her profile, or, if she gives a location, it isn't real for very obvious safety reasons.

However, if our webcammer doesn't even realize the metadata exists in the images she posts—let alone that she should scrape this information from those images for privacy reasons— she might as well post pictures of her driver's license for those who know how to mine for that additional data.

But let's say our webcammer is tech-savvy and knows to remove the metadata. What about everyone around her? What if someone else takes her picture, and that person doesn't know about the Exif data? Facial recognition is there to stand in the gap and has the ability to match the two faces—the webcammer's scraped photo to the other data-rich image—**even across platforms.**

Facebook owns Instagram, remember? Google owns YouTube. It's called the "Web" for very good reasons.

While our webcammer might take precautions, her grandmother understands only the basics of how her new iPhone works. On top of that? Grandma has no idea her granddaughter has a secret life.

This means Grandma can innocently take our gal's picture on Christmas morning then post it on Facebook to show off her family to all her friends. Facial recognition has the ability to tie our performer's real identity on Facebook to her secret identity on Instagram, as well as pinpoint the exact GPS coordinates where the photo was taken and more.

While we regular people can't access or see metadata in the images on social media, security companies can. Thus, when our webcammer applies for that real job, she could be in for a rude awakening.

Anyone trying to build a solid brand in adult entertainment has to market themselves online, usually by posting a ton of pictures. Alas, pictures have a way of coming back to bite in more ways than one.

The power of online images and how tenaciously they hang on across time underscores my point about how it's next to impossible for us to distance from our past, especially the moments we'd like most to forget. This leads into my second example. A Colorado hospital fired a medical resident when hospital employees discovered naked photos of her on the internet. The resident tried to fight back in court. She claimed she was illegally discriminated against since posing nude is not illegal, and the photos were taken before she ever worked at the hospital. In the end, though, the Colorado Court of Appeals sided with the hospital and upheld the decision to terminate the resident's employment.

According to Andrew Oh-Willeke's May 17, 2007, *Colorado News Collaborative* article, "Court: Firing Woman Due to Prior Porn Shoot Legal,":

As decided, the law in Colorado now appears to be that anyone who has ever done something in the past that might embarrass an employer when it is ultimately discovered forfeits any protection under employment

discrimination laws. People who have previously posed for porn shoots in
Colorado now bear a scarlet letter that deprives them of their legal rights
in all future jobs that they may hold. [7]

If our imaginary webcammer didn't understand just how much information her pictures were revealing, there's almost no way to escape the digital dragnet. She might be fine with low-paying entry-level positions, but most jobs with high pay, solid benefits, and healthy salaries are out of the question. The background check would automatically flag and reject her.

Perhaps she might get a good job, as we saw with the medical resident in Colorado, but she won't ever be safe. The same pictures she used to make a living by webcamming are the same pictures that can land her on welfare. All it takes is one person in the workplace to run across her pictures or content for everything to unravel.

Until we change cultural attitudes and laws, adult entertainers have no permanent way out of the industry. The same public who berates men and women for remaining in porn is the same public that forbids them to ever leave.

The Right to Be Forgotten

Pictures and metadata aren't the only links in the chains that bind. The same algorithms that can make someone a rising star in the adult entertainment industry are the same algorithms that will mark that same someone for life with a Scarlet XXX.

Between intelligent, self-evolving algorithms, data mining software, and facial recognition technology, the idea that anyone can have a secret life is ridiculous.

Big tech firms have steadfastly ignored the public outcry and summarily dismissed those who assert that people have the right to be forgotten. As it stands, everything on the internet is forever, regardless of who posted the content. It doesn't matter if someone worked in porn a year ago or forty years ago, either. Anyone who has ever done porn ever is now fair game for the Trap.

With COVID-19, most of the professional studios have been forced to close, which begs the obvious question of how they can manage to still make money in the meantime? It's simple. Film or production companies own the rights to all content forever and can legally do whatever they want with it. Unable to make new movies right now, the industry has gone back into their archives to digitize and remaster old films then released them as new content. Some of you reading might be familiar with the iconic porn film, *Debbie Does Dallas*. Though filmed in 1978, it is available online. IMDB.com even has a list of cast members. How convenient for everyone...except the actors.

Think of the implications. A teenage girl might have done some porn in the 1970s then walked away, changed her life, married, earned a degree, had a family, and built an esteemed reputation among friends and peers. But even though she is old enough to have grand-children, the Trap has breathed new life into a past she believed was long ago dead and buried. When the grandkids taught her how to post photos on Facebook, facial recognition tags her as a person she hasn't been for decades.

Since the production companies own all the rights, they can re-release old content as much as they want. They only have to pay the performers once. After that, they can do anything they want with the footage and never cut another check to the actors. Online audiences believe I am still making movies because companies remaster old footage, edit it in a different way, re-title it, and slap on a new cover before releasing it online as if it's a new film. The scenes might be five years old, but the public doesn't know that. I am constantly "releasing new movies," which is amazing since I quit filming ages ago.

The Trap doesn't care how long ago someone was in porn. The Trap doesn't care if a person willingly chose porn as a profession for a time, then decided to change their occupation or lives. The Trap doesn't care if a person chose porn out of poverty, desperation, coercion, or as a last-ditch way to survive. The Trap doesn't even care if a performer didn't choose porn at all. It only cares that the content makes money.

Maybe the woman featured in the video was secretly photographed or filmed by an unknown third party, only for that intimate act to later surface on some online porn site. Sure, the victim(s) can petition the images/videos to be taken down. But the damage is already done, and there are no guarantees the same content won't be reposted later.

There are grown women who were sexually exploited as children who, to this day, must continually petition online sites and search companies and request for the video of their rapes to be taken down...only for these videos to reemerge time and time again. Same content but new titles. The content could be posted from a new or masked IP address, by an anonymous source, or even by a complete stranger in another country.

Trying to take down content once it is live online is like playing hell's whack-a-mole and actually thinking you will win. Cyberspace is largely a lawless realm, and there are many who profit from keeping it that way. Granted, I am happy Pornhub removed a large portion of their content and no longer permits downloading. But how long were the videos they removed up and available? How many months or years could viewers freely download videos that are now banned? Once downloaded, Pornhub has no control what happens to that footage. The video has literally left the building.

Regardless how anyone ends up in adult entertainment, that performer has a fundamental human right to move on. They have the right to be forgotten. But, when it comes to those caught up in porn, technology aids and abets handing down, then enforcing, a life sentence of banishment and indefinite exploitation.

This is because pornographic content is largely responsible for making these companies the wealthiest and most powerful forces on the planet. Why would they shut down a mine with unlimited gold if they didn't have to?

The sticky nature of the World Wide Web is why I am deeply concerned for the flood of amateurs rushing to pay their bills with webcamming or performing on sites like OnlyFans. As far as I know, these online porn profiteer companies only highlight the benefits.

They tout the quick and easy money, flexible hours, and the portrayal of performers as entrepreneurs.

Remember Pornhub's Dr. Betito of the Sexual Wellness Center? "Sex has become so much less taboo that those who get a kick out of exhibitionism can do so with very little experience or equipment. The message is: anyone can be a porn star![8]"

While Dr. Betito might be correct that sex has become so much less taboo, this doesn't automatically mean sex work has become equally less taboo. The essential factor that proponents omit is that Western culture hasn't changed how it views adult performers. Our society can forgive those who watch porn, just not those who work in porn.

The prevailing sentiment appears to be that adult entertainers aren't people, rather some sort of dangerous sub-human species that should be contained, lest they cause harm to those they come in contact with. So long as sex workers remain in their place, society is fine.

No one is honestly explaining the long-term consequences of porn's short-term solutions. Companies will list all the benefits of being a performer, but when it comes to discussing how to go about leaving, there is radio silence. Potential entertainers are making life-altering decisions based on half-truths, lies of omission, or outright deception. They are led to believe they are empowered, in control, and can walk away anytime they choose, but that is only half the story. The full statement should be: "They can walk away anytime they choose, but not for long and possibly never."

For performers, the adult entertainment industry itself isn't the Trap. Rather, the layers of high-tech systems that can expose those who leave sex work, knowingly serving them up for culturally sanctioned and potentially perpetual discrimination is the Trap.

The fact that adult entertainers have no social safety net, are ineligible for government aid in times of crises, have no systems in place that offer counseling, medical care, rehabilitation, or job placement is the Trap. That morality clauses give employers the ability to fire and even blackball former sex workers is the Trap. The simple fact that places like OnlyFans require the same state or national ID to work that can be later weaponized against contributors is the Trap.

Referring again to Claire Downs' piece in *Elle*, "OnlyFans, Influencers, And the Politics of Selling Nudes During a Pandemic,":

> *Employers with morality clauses can use facial recognition software and screenshots to attach sex workers to their government names. Currently, OnlyFans requires performers to upload a driver's license for identity verification, instantly linking their content to that information.*[9]

For those who are now working in adult entertainment temporarily, I have bad news. There are already cases surfacing where women who couldn't work during COVID-19 shutdowns looked to webcamming to pay the bills and have already paid dearly. When they returned to the real job, they were summarily fired for being associated with adult entertainment. I'm not even talking about women who work with kids because, again, it shouldn't make a difference. This is legal work done by consenting adults.

Anyone who hopes to make even a decent living by webcamming has to hustle to build a name, brand, and platform using social media. This means posting pictures, images, and videos on a wide variety of social media sites such as Instagram, Twitter, YouTube, etc., as well as relentlessly promoting and marketing to gain more subscribers.

While this is an admirable endeavor that demonstrates creativity, drive, and a solid work ethic, it's unfortunately also tied to a stigmatized industry. Every piece of content posted online then becomes a potential landmine that the performer herself has planted.

Unfortunately, the digital footprints that future fans will follow to a performer's page or site will also become the indelible marks used later to track her down for exposure and expulsion. Everything she posted as a performer becomes evidence that can and will be used against her her in the court of public opinion and indefinitely.

This has had serious consequences for those who thought they would use sites like OnlyFans as a way to get by during the shutdowns, bringing me to my third example.

Kirsten Vaughn was a promising young mechanic who started webcamming to pay off student loans. In the April 20, 2020, *BuzzFeed News* article, "Her Colleagues Watched Her OnlyFans Account At Work. When Bosses Found Out, They Fired Her," journalist Otillia Steadman reports how, "Vaughn was on track to become the first woman master technician at Don Ayres Honda dealership in Fort Wayne (Indiana) when she was abruptly let go from her job after colleagues discovered her account on OnlyFans."[10]

Steadman's article relays how Vaughn's co-workers gathered to watch her videos at work then began sexually harassing her.

"'They literally would not shut up about my page,' said Vaughn. 'I begged them to not tell anybody, and they would laugh in my face and say, Ha, ha, ha, we're helping you make money. Shut up.'"[11]

When word of Vaughn's OnlyFans account reached management, those guilty of watching porn at work and then harassing Vaughn weren't disciplined. Rather, Vaughn was terminated despite a record as a model employee.[12]

Even though the company had previously praised her work and even posted videos featuring her on their Facebook page, the mere fact she was involved in adult entertainment appears to have overshadowed all her other accomplishments.

You Can Run, but You Can't Hide

Anyone trying to leave adult entertainment already has an uphill battle just getting a job. All you have to do is look at the handful of examples I have given, because they share more in common than porn. All three women lost their careers because others, i.e., porn viewers, exposed them.

This all reinforces my assertion that, even if an entertainer leaves the industry, there are bloodhounds everywhere to hunt her down and make sure she is returned to her "owners."

Earlier, I shared Pornhub's 2019 report declaring there were over

42 billion visits, making an average of 115 million visits per day. Before COVID-19, it was estimated that about 200,000 Americans could be classified as "porn addict," which is defined by Sergen's Medical Dictionary as:

> A condition that has been defined as a psychological addiction to, or dependence upon, pornography, characterised by obsessive viewing, reading, and thinking about pornography and sexual themes to the detriment of other areas of the viewer's life.[13]

Forty-million Americans regularly visit porn sites. Thirty-five percent of all internet downloads are related to pornography, and these numbers only continue to grow as our world, work, and lives shift more and more online.[14]

If a third of all downloads are pornography, what are the odds the woman or man who is retired from the adult industry will be able to remain unrecognized in everyday life?

If we think about the numbers in the beginning of the book that demonstrate the exponential growth of porn audiences, the odds of a performer being identified compound exponentially as well. If in 2019 Pornhub had over forty-two billion visits and an average of a hundred and fifteen million visits per day, what are the chances any entertainer can escape notice indefinitely?

The Trap doesn't care if a girl/woman leaves because performers are easily replaceable. The industry certainly isn't struggling to find new entertainers. New people join daily. Also remember there is also the forty-plus years of old footage sitting around just waiting to be digitized as well.

Again, my issue isn't directly with the industry, rather the aftermath and consequences for those who desire to leave and pursue a normal life and a job outside of sex work. The Trap wields the full force of the internet, the self-evolving smart algorithms that power social media, and search engines to make any escape at best temporary and at worst futile.

The Trap draws energy and power through cycles. When you look at those individuals who possess the highest probability of ending up doing some form of sex work, they overwhelmingly come from abusive backgrounds, are trying to escape a desperate situation, or a combination of both. Because of the Trap, though, entertainers only escape one cycle—abuse, poverty, powerlessness—to naively step into another cycle of exploitation, shame, and permanent exile.

As I have hopefully shown with not only my own story, but also with other cases, though there are too many to put in one book, the Trap isn't overly concerned with workers quitting. Now that we are in a digital world, everyone is interconnected through a vast global nexus that penetrates every aspect of modern life. This means that the adult industry couldn't have done better if it had put ankle monitors on every single entertainer.

Once those who work in the adult entertainment industry realize there is no way to remove the stigma of the Scarlet XXX, why not just go back into the industry? Where else are they going to go? What else can they do? Escape was an illusion, and freedom a ticking bomb. The entertainer eventually realizes what she feared is actually true. She really is trash, at least in society's eyes. And what does our society do with trash? We throw it away, burn it, or recycle it.

8

THE BOX

Welcome to solitary confinement. If the adult performer isn't isolated and trapped because of emotional damage, money, or addiction, she is trapped because what other work can she get? Or, more importantly, what other work can she keep? At this point, the entertainer probably has tried to leave only to realize that leaving was a fool's dream. What better trap than the World Wide Web? Banished and blackballed, where else can she go?

Is it any wonder sex workers have such high suicide rates?

The cycle of shame, self-hatred, and depression only continues to intensify, not only due to the nature of the work, but also because of what is required to market her content. In the last chapter, I mentioned how performers have little choice but to use the internet, social media, and email to build a following and a brand. Yet, social media, the internet, and email are open to everyone and anyone who has something to say, no matter how vile or vicious.

As adult entertainers, there comes a point we are no longer only in the cage, we are in the cage placed inside the "box." The box is wide open to everyone else for judgement and further exploitation.

We are heading deeper into the Trap and, again, I need to warn you that we are going to discuss things that people might find distressing, such as cyber-bullying, rape, stalking, murder, and suicide. But I thank you for coming this far, for being brave, and I only ask that you please continue to keep an open mind and heart.

My aim is to allow the public a different form of free and open access to insider knowledge in hopes that people might reach beyond assumptions and start asking good questions, tough questions. Certainties don't allow us to change or to improve. Only those armed with fresh insight, who are willing to learn, discuss, and engage might be able to make the world better. Regardless of any one person's opinion about porn—pro or con—the way this industry operates is not only unethical, but inhumane.

Troll Food

Even though we as performers have been shut in the box, we still have to make a living and cultivate a fan base using the internet.

Not only do outsiders have the luxury of hiding behind anonymous monikers that have little chance of being identified, but social media platforms do little to nothing to curtail hate speech or threats of violence. Our society knows cyberbullying is real, but children and young people are the priority, which is as it should be. Just because society places our youth at the top of the agenda doesn't mean adult entertainers don't deserve some place on that list. Due to the nature of our work, we attract some of the most unstable, angry, and cold-blooded followers.

Imagine being called every filthy name thinkable day in and day out every time you open Twitter or check your posts on Instagram. Picture how you might handle anonymous commenters posting the myriad of reasons you deserve to die, and then elaborating in gruesome detail all the exact ways your life should/will be snuffed out. Every time you get online, you try to ignore the people posting how they hope you are raped, tortured, and butchered, that your kids die slowly from some horrible disease, your dog dies, and so on.

Adult entertainers are human beings. How easily this seems to be forgotten.

I have been unable to fully retire as an adult performer due to the nature of the internet. Film companies recycling my old content hasn't helped, either. It's part of the Trap, and I am stuck whether I am actively working or not. I have an official work-related email I still maintain and check semi-regularly even though I have stopped performing.

Back when I was actively working, however, email was a lifeline to keep in touch with agents, producers, filmmakers, fans, etc. Like any responsible businessperson, I didn't have the luxury of ignoring messages. It could have been an email about new work or a potential job. Some messages might have been from real fans who wanted to connect and say nice things. Obviously, I wanted to write back to the kind and supportive followers and thank them. Wouldn't any celebrity, entrepreneur, or business owner want to do the same?

Yet, email is a game of Russian roulette even now that I have stopped actively performing. I have no way to discern the true content of any email until I open it. The title and preview might claim to be fan mail, when it is actually a death threat.

I have fielded countless emails from senders who, for whatever reason, felt compelled to write me long messages telling me they knew where I lived, the ways they planned to burn down my house with me and my family inside, or how they intended to break in, tie me up, then force me to watch them rape and murder my children before they raped and murdered me.

Though I could go on, I believe I have made my point. To this day, it never ceases to amaze me how inventive hateful humans can be. What can I do about it? As a porn actress, aren't I asking for it? If anyone else received the same volume of similar messages, wouldn't they have some form of recourse, or at the very least, the sympathy and compassion of others?

How many emails like this could you receive before you broke down or fell apart? What if the messages were sent to your sister, brother, partner, siblings, friends, or even your children? Would you feel they deserved it? Could you remain silent? If anyone you cared about was being trolled online the way adult entertainers are, could you dismiss it? Why is it then considered acceptable to do to us?

The Devil and The Deep Blue Sea

So, whom do we look to for help?

For the moment, let's set aside any person or entity directly related to the porn industry such as directors, producers, or even the porn sites themselves. The sites that profit from our content aren't going to protect entertainers from threats, harassment, or harm for the simple reason that they can't. It would be practically impossible. There are too many performers and too many ways we are exposed to toxic or dangerous people in an online world.

Even Hollywood can't protect mainstream movie stars and actors from crazies, so it's unrealistic to think adult entertainers would enjoy shelter that no one in regular entertainment can find either. The burden remains with the individual actor. We are on our own when it comes to dealing with trolls, stalkers, and potentially unstable or dangerous persons.

As for protecting us once we leave the adult industry, there are a handful of groups spearheading legislation to make it illegal to discriminate against adult entertainers because of our past work history. They are fighting to create laws to shield us from being fired, bullied, and threatened due to past work history. Yet, these advocacy groups who do want to protect the performers, at least from my perspective, might as well be yelling into a hurricane.

Much of the proposed legislation does more to control, criminalize, and stigmatize adult performers than to protect them.

According to the February 29, 2020, *Los Angeles Times* article "'Scarlet Letter Statute': L.A.'s Adult Performers Strike Back Against State Registry Bill," Assembly Bill 2389, dubbed by one industry attorney as a "scarlet letter statute," evoked massive backlash since the bill did nothing to combat the stigma and discrimination against adult entertainers.[1] Instead, the proposed legislation focused more on compiling a database for the purposes of proper licensing to then be used to exercise increased regulation and control:

> *AB2389 is a bill that, like SESTA/FOSTA, is dressed to look like it seeks to protect adult entertainers, when in fact, it seeks to further criminalize them,' wrote Antonia Crane, founder and director of Soldiers of the Pole, a stripper labor movement in California. 'The bill allows the state to 'register,' meaning to fingerprint, record, ID and to police, the most vulnerable workforce in the world.*[2]

It's just more chains that bind.

Even into 2020, it appears lawmakers continue to miss the point. Politicians, at least in this case, didn't even bother talking to performers or anyone who represented them. One of the major complaints about AB2389 was that those who drafted the bill didn't dedicate the time and resources needed to educate themselves about the industry, how it worked, or even about the people it would impact. As a result, lawmakers continue to fixate on the wrong issues and draft bills intended to catalogue and control the workers while turning a blind eye to the very system that keeps performers chained and holds all the keys to their locks. Government is eager to register sex workers but then fails to pass any laws that prevent future discriminatory practices.

Many adult entertainers are regular people trying to survive. Though this has always been the case on some level, the COVID-19 pandemic has revealed how many people are desperate enough to turn to working in the adult industry just to buy food and diapers. Remember Pornhub boasted they had added 98,000 new entertainers in 2019. How much higher were those numbers in 2020 with so many people out of work and unable to get government aid?

When talking about porn workers today, we are no longer referring to a fringe segment of society. Rather, the webcammers or indie porn stars might very well be neighbors, friends, or relatives who thought they had found a temporary refuge, a way to make it through a financial storm, only to fall prey to a lie.

There is no longer any such thing as working temporarily in the adult industry, especially if lawmakers persist on trying to register them. Many advocacy groups argue that mandating government licenses and registration would only force sex work deeper underground, leaving performers more defenseless than ever. Any entertainer trying to retire might as well forfeit all hope of a real job should she be in possession of such a license. AB2389, had it passed, would actually have made it easier for potential employers to discriminate against adult entertainers. Why hire security companies to comb social media when a business can simply check if a candidate is or has ever been registered as a sex worker?

Why would a state create a database of those who have done nothing illegal and make them register as if they are convicted sex offenders? The bigger question we might want to ask is why aren't they proposing a similar database to register those who own and run porn sites and the businesses that advertise on those platforms?

FREE Flesh, Big Money

In the pre-digital age, consumers had to pay directly to view/consume porn. They had to buy or subscribe to magazines and pay to purchase or rent movies. Those who created porn, including the actors, made money off royalties. Pornographers relied on royalties from the number of films, videos, calendars, etc., sold.

Models and performers don't make royalties off pornographic content. We've pretty much always been paid a flat fee for the print or film. Ah, but should one get big enough, there were once other ways of generating more income. Models and actors could make royalties on certain items sold in stores. For instance, a famous Playboy Bunny or a big-name porn actress could offer her own line of sexy costumes for the bedroom.

This all changed with the digital age. When porn shifted from glossy magazine paper and videotapes to blips of 0s and 1s, an entirely new economic model emerged. In the early years, viewers had to pay sites if they wanted to watch porn, but this limited profit for obvious reasons. Since a person can't pay cash to an online site like they could at video store or adult shop, viewers had to use a credit card. But credit cards leave a paper trail, and this created a barrier. Plenty of people might have been willing to fork out cash for a *Playboy* or *Penthouse* magazine or buy a porn DVD with cash because they could keep it a secret. There was a much smaller percentage of people who didn't care if porn sites showed up on the credit card bill than those who cared...a lot. Married men and those in positions of power or authority who risked backlash, made up a lot of the cash consumer base. Also, back then, not everyone had a credit card. Going online actually risked substantially shrinking porn viewership.

The sites needed more eyes to make bigger profits but charging viewers clearly shackled expansion. What could these sites do to ensure online porn would not only grow, but also grow exponentially?

Make it free.

Herein lies the problem, though. There is no such thing as free. Sites who offer free porn still have to make money. The servers, band-width, engineers, site managers, and the many other employees who run the porn machine twenty-four hours a day, seven days a week, have to be paid. How could these sites not only cover their costs, but also make a profit if the product they were offering cost the viewer nothing?

Advertising.

Outside third parties ended up funding the entire operation and continue to do so now more than ever. Companies are making fortunes off of the adult industry. Many of these businesses outsource marketing and advertising to agencies. Advertising and marketing firms compete for business by showcasing the results of successful campaigns, and success is measured in large part by the smartest media buys that get the product in front of the most eyes and convert views to clicks to sales. Companies trust that their advertising/mar-keting people are helping them earn profits legally, which they are.

And, as I have said time and time again, a lot of porn is legal.

Technically, the advertising/marketing departments and agencies aren't doing anything against the law by placing media buys with porn sites. Also, since porn is widely accepted as a socially acceptable vice/private activity, especially for men, these companies aren't even doing anything wrong, especially if that is the target demographic for the product. They are doing their job, which is to connect potential consumers with their product/service in the most efficient and profitable way.

From a marketer's perspective, short of a Super Bowl commercial, where else outside of free porn could a firm reliably count on millions or even hundreds of millions of eyes encountering their ad? In some ways porn is even better than the Super Bowl. After all, the Super Bowl happens once a year and a 30-second ad buy can cost upwards of one million dollars, but online porn runs three hundred sixty-five days a year, and a million-dollars buys a hell of a lot of website ads. It is just a sound business strategy.

Even though brands, businesses, and corporations indirectly finance free access to the entertainers, they are conveniently not directly responsible for any harm that results from this business model. They are content to enjoy the financial windfall. What happens to the performer, her ability to leave the industry, or to get a real job, isn't part of the equation.

In the beginning of this book, I mentioned the strict regulations placed on the tobacco and alcohol industries. They're severely limited when it comes to advertising. As the result of legislation, magazines, television, billboards, sporting events, etc., were all deemed off-limits. The United States legal system took great pains to also make certain these industries were unable to sell to or even influence minors. But where is the regulation for online ads to porn sites? Where are the restrictions? It isn't okay for a tobacco company to finance a racing team, or a tequila company to bankroll a sports team, but somehow, we seem to stop asking questions when it comes to a vast array of companies who finance free porn.[3] Most of us don't ask questions because we don't even know that we need to, and that's a problem.

From my perspective, it looks a lot like a case of "rules for thee and not for me."

Tobacco and alcohol companies can't market in ways that attract minors. Remember Joe Camel? According to the Federal Trade Commission's statement released on May 28, 1997, "Joe Camel Advertising Campaign Violates Federal Law," the FTC Says:

> *The Joe Camel advertising campaign violates federal law, the Federal Trade Commission charged today. The campaign, which the FTC alleges was successful in appealing to many children and adolescents under 18, induced many young people to begin smoking or to continue smoking cigarettes and as a result caused significant injury to their health and safety. The FTC charged that R.J. Reynolds Tobacco Company, the seller of Camel cigarettes, promoted an addictive and dangerous product through a campaign that was attractive to those too young to purchase cigarettes legally. In fact, the FTC said, after the campaign began the percentage of kids who smoked Camels became larger than the percentage of adults who smoked Camels.*[4]

Not only is the box free and open to adults who want to watch, there is no mandate for these sites or the companies funding them to prevent minors from peering inside as well. There are no guidelines forbidding the type of ads that could possibly attract children, as was the case with Joe Camel and R.J. Reynolds. There are no penalties for supplying a supposedly restricted product to an underage audience.

We have entire government agencies that police and regulate tobacco, alcohol, firearms, and other restricted products. Meanwhile, online porn is the uncomfortable elephant in the room no one seems willing to address. Government entities remain committed to fingerprinting and cataloguing porn stars for the purposes of stricter regulation. But while they fixate on the performer or product, there is no similar fixation on those who finance and distribute the product. If we follow through with the metaphor, what would happen to a tobacco or alcohol company that provided minors all the cigarettes and booze they wanted for free?

When it comes to online access to porn, the burden is shifted to the parents and guardians. It's their fault for not watching their kids, for failing to set up enough parental controls, even though we will see later these parental controls are laughably flimsy.

Jane & Jack-in-The-Box

Whether one is pro-porn or anti-porn, does it seem just that the only ones shackled are the performers? Companies can move on and advertise elsewhere. Audiences enjoy total anonymity and even a degree of social sanction. Anyone anywhere with internet access can watch the entertainer dance in the box, including minors, but those inside the box are never and will never be free.

Please understand that my goal here isn't to shame anyone who has ever watched free online porn. I have spent most of my adult life as an object of scorn and derision. I understand at a fundamental level how bad it feels to be scolded and humiliated. I only mention this new business model of how free porn is financed in order to open your eyes to just how powerful the Trap is and how, thus far, it operates largely unseen and unchecked.

These corporations and brands are advertising legally. Again, a lot of porn isn't illegal, and many people see nothing wrong with adult entertainment. This said, how many average investors even know all this is going on? How many regular people with 401Ks, IRA accounts, or a small stock portfolio realize they are inadvertently financing free porn? Maybe they would be okay with it, maybe not. But shouldn't they at least be aware?

We, as a society, vote our conscience with our dollars. Doesn't it then seem only reasonable to ask for transparency, for companies to disclose the places and ways they advertise to consumers as well as investors? And if companies want to continue using this advertising/marketing model, that is their call. But those who purchase their goods and services or invest in those companies' stocks should ideally have a say, too.

Perhaps with greater awareness, companies and consumers

could do more to make necessary changes in the industry. Performers could leave without penalty. We could remove the Scarlet XXX, and porn would be held to the same standards as comparable industries.

Alone in the Crowd

Adult entertainers, shunned by the outside world, remain isolated. We don't even really have community within our own industry. By and large, those in the adult entertainment business don't create community for many reasons. Namely, we can't.

Thus, far, I have covered the most common areas of adult entertainment—stripping, webcamming, escorting, and porn. Obviously, one of the first reasons those in sex work have historically struggled to create any sort of strong internal community is because everyone is in direct competition with each other.

If you are an exotic dancer, this is an extremely competitive job. Every girl wants to be a Night Girl with a long list of whales for clients. What is the incentive to bond with another dancer who might take her spot or steal her best customers? The same thing goes for those in escorting. For the escort, having a long list of dependable clients who pay big money is her lifeline. It's in her interest to be extremely territorial and guard that list because those clients pay the rent.

Those who remain in the Trap long enough can become too broken and too ashamed to forge even simple friendships. To make money and remain relevant, performers have to do as many jobs as they can. Every time they are on set, a call, or on a screen, a small fragment of their humanity crumbles until there is nothing left but dust. This systematically erodes their ability to trust, which is a core ingredient of almost all relationships.

They can't date like regular people for the same reasons they can't get and hold regular jobs. They are banned from the very social circles where they might even meet a partner who isn't in the industry or obsessed by it. Even should a performer meet a nice guy or gal, what happens when that person finds out what they really do for a living?

Any partner is risking a Scarlet XXX by association. If the public finds out a corporate executive's wife used to be a porn star, what then? What about an elementary school teacher outed for dating a former webcammer or a politician married to an escort? The fallout for the partner could range from being the center of the gossip mill to being shunned by friends, family and associates, to flat out risking one's career. It takes a brave, secure person to be willing to share the shame, so to speak.

And should there be some rare occasion a performer found someone who would treat them as a person and without judgement, who is willing to take any heat that might come, would it matter? No. Sadly, it wouldn't matter for a number of reasons.

Often, the performer's ability to create any kind of emotional bond is too damaged. She cannot truly believe the person could love her and would push them away. Every moment, she is bracing for her partner to turn on her and throw her out. Why not be first to walk away? If she really does love the other person, she knows the best way to show she cares is to end the relationship before the other person suffers consequences of her Scarlet XXX.

Continually isolated, the psychological, emotional, and physical toll for the entertainer escalates. To remain sane, performers steadily retreat further and further inside themselves. They compartmentalize so they can play the part that keeps fans happy—bubbly, fun, sexy—but it's all an act. The performer is a puppet starring in her own tragedy. By now, you are familiar with the routine, how most entertainers rely more and more on drugs, alcohol, and prescriptions just to make it through the day. Additionally, once they realize they are unlikely to escape, they are now desperate to do everything they can in order to remain a valuable commodity in the one profession left open to them. Not only are they aging, but viewers are craving increasingly extreme body types.

To keep making money, many performers will turn to plastic surgery. They can get larger breasts, bigger lips, a larger butt, smaller waist, tanning injections, fillers, etc. When they started out, they might have been a naturally pretty or even beautiful girl. By some point, however, due to audience demands, the entertainer can end up a walking anime character or worse, a freak show.

Before, she couldn't get a regular job because algorithms and search engines singled her out for discrimination. After a certain point, her own face and body will betray her. Who will hire a woman with 32FFF breasts for anything but a job in adult entertainment? She could earn a Harvard law degree or a PhD in aeronautical engineering, and it wouldn't make any difference.

Many entertainers are having surgeries to literally look like Barbie. Women augment their breasts to sizes so large they have to travel to countries like Brazil, which has no restrictions on the breast augmentation size, because no responsible surgeon would agree to implant to the size of a 32S. If she can keep the viewers staring at the largest breasts in the world, they won't ever look at her face and notice the faint-but-relentless signs she is aging, despite the injections and Botox. Some of these surgeries are to keep the fans happy, but remember, she is a mess inside and has been conditioned to loathe herself. This is why severe body dysmorphia is so common.

At this point, the performer is a physical and emotional train wreck trapped in an industry that will only set her free once she is no longer profitable, and maybe not even then. Without community, compassion, or even legislation to help her, the downward spiral continues into a living hell.

9

MEET MS. MEAT

Full disclosure: this section will possibly be the hardest to read, because the truth is often ugly, overwhelming, or downright terrifying. I will warn you ahead of time that this chapter contains graphic descriptions of disturbing content. But I have gone to great lengths to filter these accounts down to only what details are necessary to support my points.

This section is the worst-case-scenario for the adult entertainer, when she is unable to leave the porn industry. Our society's unquenchable hunger for porn has thus far taken priority over everything, including the wellbeing of the performers who feed that need.

Like the Venus flytrap, the Trap's prime directive is to survive and spread. The Trap lives to consume and consumes to live. The most immediate source of sustenance are naturally those in the adult industry. Baited with promises and lured with lies, many performers end up trapped only to be devoured and slowly dissolved and digested as fuel.

You might be asking yourself, "Where is the hope in all this?"

The adult entertainment industry, in and of itself, is not the Trap. Rather it is the layers of algorithmic chains, the search engine search lights, digital dogs and social circle sentinels that make certain no one who enters ever leaves. Or, if they do, it isn't for long. The Trap can only continue to exist if we allow it. Even with all the online chains, doors, locks, barriers, and alarms, these matter only if we as a culture continue to dehumanize performers, refusing reentry into the "normal" world outside of adult entertainment.

Keeping in mind human nature and our hard-wired biological drive to reproduce, it's foolish to believe we could ever shut down adult entertainment. There are those who would argue we shouldn't want to shut it down because censorship has a nasty way of getting out of control, meaning we could potentially spiral in another, equally destructive direction. Regardless of preference or opinion, the fact remains that sex work is the oldest profession in the world for good reasons. Even though adult entertainment will always be around, it doesn't automatically mean the Trap can't be ripped up by the roots. We, as a society, have the power to dismantle the Trap. But we can't fight what we won't face.

The Outer Limits: Porn and Purgatory

Banished from mainstream society and with no legal safeguards against discrimination, many adult performers have no choice but to return to porn. This section is about the darkest corners of pornography, the outer limits where almost anything goes. We have toured all the other levels and have now reached the adult entertainer's final destination.

In short, this is the place where porn stars go to die.

When we explored the porn cage, I talked about how too many young and naive women end up victims of bait-and-switch schemes. The first of those bait-and-switch scams is often a webcammer who was never given the choice to take part in porn films. Rather, someone else made the choice for her.

The *Guardian* article, "A rough trade: Martin Amis reports from the high-risk, increasingly violent world of the pornography industry," includes a series of candid interviews with various members of the porn industry. A porn star by the name of "Temptress," relayed a frighteningly real and all too common scenario for many in our industry:

> *Some girls are used in nine months or a year. An 18-year-old, sweet young thing, signs with an agency, makes five films in her first week. Five directors, five actors, five times five: she gets phone calls. A hundred movies in four months. She's not a fresh face anymore. Her price slips and she stops getting phone calls. Then it's, 'Okay, will you do anal? Will you do gang bangs?' Then they're used up. They can't even get a phone call. The market forces of this industry use them up.*[1]

Once in the porn industry, another bait-and-switch tactic exacts a terrible price on the actors. Instead of progressing from milder adult films and building a fan following that would give a performer power to say no, too many entertainers are unwittingly fast-tracked into the extreme films. They are preyed on by opportunists, which is nothing new.

And, what is considered extreme is also changing.

Remember how the 1980s that Vanessa Williams, the first black Miss America, was also the first Miss America to hand back her crown?[2] Two years before the scandal, Williams, while working as a makeup artist and receptionist at a modeling agency, agreed to pose for risqué photos. According to the *Time Magazine* article "The Scandal that Cost Miss America Her Crown,":

> *The photographer had assured her at the time, she told People, that the photos were merely silhouettes, in which she'd be unidentifiable and that they would never leave the studio. But they did leave the studio, partly because she was identifiable: photos of Miss America in compromising positions, some of them involving another nude woman, were worth their weight in gold.*[3]

Playboy declined to purchase the images even though they had been given the first bid. Not only did *Playboy* refuse to buy the photos, but founder and owner Hugh Hefner ironically denounced

Penthouse Magazine's subsequent publication of Williams' nude photos as "immoral" and "improper."

> *"'The single victim in all of this was the young woman herself, whose right to make this decision was taken away from her,' TIME quoted Hefner as saying. 'If she wanted to make this kind of statement, that would be her business, but the statement wasn't made by her.'"*[4]

Here we see a good example of a young, naive woman trusting a photographer's word. She made very little money from the shoot and was flat out lied to then later exploited. What made the *Penthouse* pictures so controversial was less that Williams posed nude and far more that she did so with another woman in lesbian scenarios. Anyone over a certain age can probably recall the public losing its collective mind about the obscene and lewd...lesbian material. Women having sexual relations with other women was simply beyond the pale and too perverse.

For today's porn viewer, girl-on-girl action is considered only slightly racier than watching a man and woman having sex. It's so common as to be regarded as mild or tame in the porn world. What was extreme in the 1980s, 1990s, or even ten years ago, is now normal. Today, all one has to do is glance at the most searched for terms and take note of the videos with millions of views. Even Pornhub boasted how the search term 'amateur' was so prevalent that it all but defined 2019.

Along the outer limits of porn, viewers look for videos with scenarios featuring incest (not the step-family type), rape, kidnapping, torture, pseudo-bestiality, sci-fi space alien sex, and mock 'snuff' films. Sex with grannies, midgets, midget grannies, the morbidly obese, amputees, ugly chicks and more. Viewers want to gawk at rosebuds, scat films, golden showers (urination and incontinence), glory holes (walls where only the bottom end of a woman is exposed, her legs restrained so long lines of strangers can have sex through a hole in the plywood without ever seeing her face), and more.

What really saddens me is that so many of the categories exploit the elderly, the damaged, and the weak, serving their misfortune up as entertainment. It might not disturb me as deeply if the performers were afforded some amount of dignity, but the video titles and ads are demeaning, dehumanizing, and flat out cruel. For example, senior citizens who can't cover their bills with that Social Security check are signing up to bare it all for those who want to watch. I'm not here to judge their decision to do porn or judge those who watch. But when online ads announce, "Watch Desperate Grannies Suck," or "Giant Granny Orgy," or "Teen Virgin's Step-Granny Shows Him the Ropes?" It's degrading and death by search keyword.

These ads and titles sound more like a carnie crowing for crowds to come watch a freak show. But that is what the outer limits makes performers into: freaks.

Dehumanization and Desensitization

Many viewers have long since lost their fascination and zeal for conventional anal sex. No, they want double and triple anal, or triple-vaginal at the same time as double-anal, or double vaginal at the same time as double anal. The more the performer's physical limits can be pushed to frightening extremes, the more viewers log on and line up to gape at "gaping" until even this is boring to them, and they demand something wilder, crazier, bigger!

The actress, meanwhile, suffers large groups of men brutalizing her body at the same time. Though she will suffer permanent injury, she has to play her role convincingly if she wants to keep working, attract more viewers, followers, fans, etc. The business model practically demands her to continually up the ante until she is venturing into the depraved and dangerous. Gang bang competitions are a good example. Yes, I know I just hit hyperdrive, but gang bang competitions really are a thing.

Yes, you read that correctly: gang bang competitions.

American porn star, Lisa Sparxxx set a world record by having sex with 919 men in a single day during Eroticon 2004, a Polish convention that was part of the Third Annual World Gangbang Championship.[5] Sparxxx outpaced the former record-holders who had *only* managed to have sex with 646 men in 2002, and again with 759 in 2003.[6] Sparxxx has set the goal of having sex with a thousand men in twenty-four hours, but, like the record-holders before her, she, too, had to stop because she was bleeding, crying and in too much pain to go on. Like the other women, she also had to be whisked away for emergency medical care. This last part, however, you might not find mentioned on any site covering these events. They fixate on the sex while editing out the sutures.

Keep in mind the year: 2004. In 1984, the most extreme pornography most people could conceive of was lesbian scenarios. There were, of course, seedy underground pornographers who proffered the extreme content, but this was a realm relegated to a rare slice of society and an extremely niche audience. This type of content was a million miles from anything one might discover in the areas of mainstream porn. Twenty years later, however, a single woman breaks a world record by publicly having sex with almost one thousand men in under twenty-four hours.

I would also like you to keep in mind that this record was, as I write this, set almost twenty years ago. If the definition of extreme could shift from the twenty years separating 1984 to 2004 so drastically, what is it like now? In a word: a nightmare.

Gang bang films where one girl is passed around and ravaged by ten, fifteen, thirty men in one film aren't uncommon. Not just large groups of men with a single girl, but men with unnaturally large penises crammed into the same places at the same time with that girl. One actress might be having sex with six men at a time (you know, the ol' triple-vaginal combined with triple anal act) while she has a penis shoved down her throat and a penis in each hand, making it technically nine men at the same time. Meanwhile other males might be masturbating, ejaculating all over her while the other men take their turns. They could also be slapping her, shaming her, and calling her names until one of the men finishes, and another tormentor can slip in and take over. This can go on for an hour or even longer. In fact, the longer "the slut" can last, the more abuse she endures, the more viewers this video will attract. Which is great for the site who rakes in the cash, but the girl? She only makes whatever she was initially paid for this sort of abuse. Oh, and trust me that the hour-long video, provided it is legal, took at least a day to make.

And, if you recall from earlier, videos such as these have only recently been vetted, meaning a girl in a scenario might not have been paid at all. It could have been an actual attack someone filmed then uploaded. Porn distribution sites, however, have historically done little to no policing and/or vetting and why would they? They made big bucks from advertisers, and a film that extreme was a sure hit for a ton of views. Whether or not a young woman really was the victim of a crime was beside the point.

All this said, the goal of success sets a capitalist cascade in motion, a race to the bottom for the most eyes and the most money. If this video attracted wide attention, thus making a ton of money, then the next logical step is to outdo the performance the next time, and the next, and so on.

In these videos, the woman doesn't always have to pretend to enjoy what is happening to her. She might be legitimately screaming, crying, struggling, and fighting for her life. Men bind her, gag her, and have their way, tossing her around like a rag doll while she begs for mercy.

Videos that feature violent acts against women are becoming so popular that we, as a society, would be wise to be very, very concerned. Performers are tied up, choked, slapped, punched, whipped, beaten, and hooked up to batteries and shocked, all while male performers shove penises, fists, dildoes, or giant foreign objects anywhere they can find—or make—an opening.

Just How Bad Is It?

I have already listed out the warnings for what is ahead. Feel free to skip this section and move to the next chapter. Frankly, I would like to skip ahead, too, but we are in a crisis, and only the unvarnished truth might divert us off this self-destructive course that is erasing our empathy and overwriting our humanity. I particularly want those who are unfamiliar with porn to know just how extreme the field is becoming, at least providing enough details to appreciate the performer's living hell that is free for anyone to watch...children included.

As an adult entertainer, I have gone out of my way to avoid extreme porn professionally, though not always successfully. Yet, even my most nightmarish experiences can't compare. Being in the industry, I was obviously aware these films and fetishes existed, but I already had enough garbage in my head and didn't need to go looking for more, that is until I finally decided to write this book. To write about the Trap and impress on readers the appalling shifts in the type of content lumped into the content on mainstream porn sites, I had to watch.

Take my word for it: some things you simply can never unsee. As hardened as I believed I had become, these films reduced me to tears. I hope I can sketch out the idea enough for you to appreciate the true gravity of the situation.

Ms. Meat

Again, a warning that this section includes graphic description of torture, sexual acts, and verbal and emotional abuse.

One particularly disturbing trend involves films where females are reduced to animals: dairy cows to be specific. There are countless videos that use this fetish, and all of them horrified me. There is one particular video that seems to be among the most popular, and it is over an hour long. I won't reveal the name because I don't want to advertise for it. But this video managed to combine all the worst of what is becoming trendy, so I will give you a bare-bones summary.

The movie begins with an opening shot of at least five naked women locked in a variety of tiny outdoor cages fixed into a hillside. One woman is trapped in the ground with only her head visible through a hole in the trapdoor.

The camera pans over, and three gagged women, bound with

ropes and chains, teeter on a contraption remnant of what was once called the *cavaletto squarciapalle*, also known as the wooden horse.[7]

Historically, this device was used as a form of punishment and is where we get the modern expression, "To run someone out of town on a rail." The condemned party was forced to straddle a thick, triangular wooden beam with the point at the top directly under the crotch. This was not only painful, but could do permanent damage if prolonged over time, especially when the powers in charge added weights to the victim's legs.[8]

The skit clearly took its inspiration from historical torture methods. All three women are rigged into a contraption that uses gravity to force each woman to do some act—balance on tiptoes, not move, keep a head up despite exhaustion and agony to redistribute weight —or the others suffer since all their actions/or inactions are connected. For instance, so long as one woman on the right remains standing on her tiptoes (barefoot and in mud to make it more difficult), she can alleviate pressure on the woman strapped nude to the wooden horse. She can only remain on her tiptoes so long though. Eventually she cannot help but grow weary.

Every time she stumbles or tries to take a break, her body weight pulls down on the woman strapped to the wooden horse, thus gouging her naked groin. It's all very complex, tortuous and chilling. No matter what any one woman does, one of the others will suffer while she struggles to ward off exhaustion. The camera operator keeps zooming in on the women's tear-streaked eyes filled with panic and pain, while the other girls keep mumbling, "I'm sorry," to one another.

The next scene features some hidden master marching these women, naked, barefoot and bound with chains through a forest. Some have their hands locked in pillory boards. The blonde from the scene I just described marches chained like the others, but a *cavaletto squarciapalle* is chained between her legs so that every step inflicts even more pain and injury to her groin.

The camera again focuses on the desperate eyes and smeared makeup, or zooms in to show the rough, rocky terrain these women must walk barefoot over. Eventually, the women are herded to a barn.

The scene shifts and focuses on one woman. Coaxed like a trained dog, she obediently allows a man to clamp her into a metal apparatus that looks like a prop out of a bad horror movie.

Once immobile, he gags her, then hooks her up to a mechanical milking machine that pumps her breasts while the man keeps calling her his "cow." He proceeds to do everything imaginable and unimaginable to this helpless woman, calling her names, then coaching her to tell him—or, rather, acknowledge with a moan or grunt—how much she likes what is being done to her.

I had to stop watching, I was so upset. Besides, I think that is more than enough to illustrate what is out there and available with a few clicks.

This is only one of many films where women are caged, coached to violate each other with broomsticks, metal rods, you name it. Women chained, gagged, abused, tossed in shallow graves, shocked with electricity, penetrated by machines, and so on. It's a bottomless pit of porn despair.

But who cares? She is a slut and deserves it. She signed up for it. She probably even loves it! Besides, she is no longer a person...she is meat.

Suffice to say, the more the actresses are violated, the better the entertainment value. This sort of torture as entertainment happens, of course, to males as well. I am by no means ignoring this group, but I do find it difficult to authentically speak for them. That and, statistically speaking, women so disproportionately represent the performers cast as victims in rape, gang bang, gang rape, and generally humiliating and violent scenarios that they constitute a majority of those physically and emotionally harmed. Any males cast as victims in similar films would suffer in much the same way.

All humans feel pain, regardless of gender.

Pound of Flesh

The damage to the body is severe. Women in their early twenties are suffering severe anal prolapsing, which is when their intestines are literally falling out of their anuses, and this is the popular fetish I previously referred to as a *rosebud*.

Many young women who are barely old enough to legally buy alcohol now have to wear adult diapers because the work has rendered them permanently incontinent. Viewers want to see films of increasingly critical anal prolapses and of women unable to maintain bladder control.

Other performers are directed to lick or suck on a distended bowel (the rosebud), opening them up to a long list of infections and illnesses, some of which can be deadly. I'm talking about parasitic infections such as giardia, bacterial infections like chlamydia and MRSA, as well as other serious STDs such as syphilis, hepatitis, HIV, just to name a few.

As someone with a nursing degree, I'm very aware of these dangers, but one doesn't necessarily have to be among the ranks of trained medical personnel to know this is bad. Those of us in what would be considered the professional porn industry understand the importance of regular testing for disease, and I can say that most professionals take testing very seriously. We have to. Sex is our business and our livelihood, but it's also our life.

There are also certain kinds of scenes professionals handle with great care. For example, many porn stars commonly perform anal sex scenes. What the audience doesn't necessarily understand is that the performer has probably done two or three enemas before the filming ever begins in order to clean out the colon and remove as much fecal matter as possible. Taking time to clean out the lower intestine minimizes the chance of contracting bacterial infections or catching a parasite.

Viewers are also misled in that they are oblivious to what really happens when the cameras stop rolling. All they see are the staged interviews where the entertainers act like we just had the best sex of our lives, something we are obviously paid (and occasionally forced) to say. They don't witness that performer writhing in pain and bleeding afterwards due to rectal or vaginal tearing, or because their intestines are damaged and falling out of their anus. There are some extreme porn companies where the performers just expect filming will be followed by a trip to the hospital and a month of recovery time.

What about the amateurs jumping onto the online porn band-wagon who are simply mimicking what they have seen in videos? They lack any understanding about the protocols in place to make these sexual acts as sterile and safe as possible. Because of this igno-rance, they don't comprehend the risks of switching from anal sex to vaginal to oral because the videos they watch have been edited to make the sexual event appear seamless. For instance, they don't know that, in between an anal sex scene and an oral sex scene, the performers took a break to wash and perhaps perform another enema. Most disturbingly, what about the injuries that viewers, particularly young viewers, might inflict or endure because they are emulating what they are seeing online? What infections or diseases could they be unwittingly catching or spreading?

While viewers might get a thrill out of watching double anal, double vaginal, double anal with double vaginal, or any of these extreme combinations, it is a very different world for the performer. Repeated trauma exacts a terrible price. It can create anal or vaginal cysts, abscesses, or even fistulas. Fistulas form when an abscess goes unnoticed or untreated. The infected pocket grows until the pressure finally punches a hole in the tissue that separates the bowel and vaginal wall so the abscess can drain. Or the abscess can break, releasing bacteria into the bloodstream that infects other organs like the heart and brain, which can be fatal. These tears or fistulas then permit fecal matter into the vagina, causing tremendous short-term and long-term damage and can lead to sterility, chronic infections, and even death. Consistent vaginal trauma can also lead to tears from the bladder into the vaginal passage so that urine pours out of the vaginal opening.

But the show must go on.

And though it would be fantastic if all the porn companies followed the safety rules to the letter, the truth is some don't. While the actors might take disease and infections seriously, sometimes we have no choice but to do as we are told if we want to work and remain in the good graces of those who hold the power to cast us (or not) in future films. Performers slated to film might have an STD or vaginal infection, but it doesn't matter. There are directors who will order a performer with a herpes outbreak to slather concealer over open sores and get back to work. I know this because I have witnessed it more times than I care to admit. The industry will claim they would never allow anyone to perform who had any disease or infection, and the viewing public has no way of knowing any different.

All along, the viewers believe this is all consensual and that the adult entertainer is having the time of her life. She isn't really crying or begging, it's an act. What they don't know, or perhaps don't care to know is that performers are regularly victimized and have no recourse. Performers are routinely raped on set or forced into having sex if they want the job or to be paid for the film that they just survived making. Producers, directors, camera crews all get a piece, and her willingness to cooperate is immaterial.

Who will believe a "nymphomaniac" has been raped?

There have been cases where independent investigators collected actual evidence of rape and sexual assault. But even after providing irrefutable evidence to the film company that a producer, director, or crew member is guilty of serial rape, the companies refused to take any action to protect their performers. These abusers are left to continue assaulting young women and men.

Not only is the performer helpless against her employers, but the films have created a false reality for fans. She is now a target everywhere she goes because some crazy follower actually believes she enjoys being savagely raped by total strangers. If she happens to be raped, the police might take a report, but odds are better than good that no prosecuting attorney is going to take on a case that is all but unwinnable from the start.

Hey, he saw it in her videos. She was really into it.

With no advocate and no support system, the performer turns inward on herself even more. Self-harm, substance abuse, then frequently suicide. Is the film company worried? Are the online porn sites concerned? Nope. Her films live on long after she is gone. With the Trap, even death doesn't get in the way of a long porn career.

The internet is teeming with desperate young people who have no idea how the industry really works and how little agency they will have once part of the machine. Worst of all, they have no clue the Trap even exists, and that once they step through that door and the locks are in place, escape is impossible.

But no big deal.

The industry simply baits the hook, waits for a nibble, and replaces the used-up/dead performer just like the last one, and the one before, and the one before...

PART II

10

YOU ARE NOT IN CONTROL

P lot twist! Up to this point, we have focused almost solely on one side of the story: the perspective of the performer. Yet, as the saying goes, "It takes two to tango." What about the audience, those who view porn? Exactly what is happening on the other side of the screen?

I cannot emphasize this enough. The Trap is a parasitic species that has evolved with no natural predators and is wholly unique to the digital age. Though the Trap devours performers, it is actually those who watch online porn are the Trap's richest food source. Surprise!

Much of what we will be discussing in this second part of the book you can read about in far greater detail in Harvard professor Shoshana Zuboff's powerhouse book, *The Age of Surveillance Capitalism: The Fight for a Human Future at the New Frontier of Power*[1]. I will be using a lot of her research, as well as the expertise of other industry experts, scientists, researchers, psychologists, and more as we go along.

The point of everything in this book is to make you aware and educate you all in an effort that you might be more vigilant. Suffice to say, there is a hidden market that is using our online activity solely to their own advantage, regardless of what happens to those on the other side of the screen. This is called surveillance capitalism.[2]

Surveillance capitalism is a new business model, unique to the digital age. This new form of capitalism is threaded all throughout the web. It's also a primary financial engine powering online adult entertainment and strengthening the Trap.

The Trap impacts all of us, now more than ever. Yes, even those who don't watch porn. The Trap has grown so vast in such a short time that we might very well be on the verge of no return.

For those of consenting age who still want to enjoy adult entertainment, that is a personal decision, but to reiterate, adult entertainment can exist without the Trap. It is very complex, but this strangle-vine has had decades to wend itself throughout the World Wide Web. It will take time to unravel this tangled mess where it makes sense why the Trap is so insidious. I am here to tell you what should probably be on a warning label if such a label existed.

In any market system, we generally assume we are in an equitable relationship with those who provide a product or service. Over roughly the past twenty years, though, the relationship between provider and consumer has changed drastically. When it comes to online porn viewers, the adult entertainment industry is less fair and equitable trade and more, as Shoshana Zuboff would call it, a "Faustian bargain."[3]

I am not naive. Adult entertainment will always be around, just like humans will always want their cigarettes and alcohol. Just because we keep those substances legal and accessible doesn't automatically mean these industries don't have to play by some rules. Same with porn. I am certainly no advocate of censorship, but just because adult entertainment remains an option, that doesn't mean we must automatically serve up our souls and give this industry free rein.

Eyes Wide Shut

For a long time, I was too caught up in my own traumas to see beyond myself and realize I wasn't the only one in pain. Over time, though, as I matured and interacted more with fans who were surprisingly also struggling, I started to question everything I assumed to be true about pornography. It soon became apparent I was only seeing a small slice of a vast reality. Once I realized the big picture of how the Trap preys on performers and audiences, everything—and I mean *everything*—changed.

To be fully transparent, and it pains me to admit this, I held onto resentment and anger for years. I couldn't wrap my head around why so many men were not only watching porn, but also becoming consumed by it. How could they be like my ex-husband and jeopardize their jobs, relationships, finances, reputations, and families for...this? More importantly, why were men suddenly craving darker, rougher, and more perverse and violent scenarios? As a performer, I found myself viewing the audience the same way they viewed me. They weren't human. I hardened myself. If they wanted to take advantage of me, then that could go both ways. I could take advantage of them, too.

Hey, I promised to be honest.

But this ate away at me. I couldn't live with myself. I loathed this feeling. We were all humans and shouldn't be preying on each other. It wasn't right. We weren't enemies. At least we shouldn't be, right? Yet, this is a common knee-jerk reaction whenever we as a society try to have any discussion about porn. Folks tend to quickly take sides, oversimplifying an extremely complex reality into us versus them. I mentioned this dynamic in the beginning of this book. One side blames the entertainers for creating pornographic content. The other side rails against the audience for consuming porn and driving pornographic content deeper into darker territories.

This is the big lie, though.

As absurd as this might sound, **the performers and the viewers are actually on the same side.** The porn star and the porn viewer are both hapless pawns, pitted against the Trap. The Trap is a perverted form of capitalism's "invisible hand" and is made up of profit-making powers deploying self-evolving algorithms that maximize earnings from online porn.[4] The Trap is moving entertainers *and* viewers around a board they can't see in a game they can't win because no one even knows such a game exists.

It was once easy to write off porn viewers. That was until I started researching and understanding how unseen forces were manipulating them, using their biology and brains against them, and profiting off their very human weaknesses without their knowledge or consent. Imagine my shock when I fully grasped that porn audiences were being exploited, too. Just like the naive performer believes she is in control, so does the person who clicks on that free porn. Ironically, the viewers are key to the Trap namely because viewers exceedingly outnumber performers, and, because of that, they are ultimately a lot more valuable.

We are going to look at the viewers because there is an old adage that, if you want to get to the heart of any problem, what do you do?

Follow the money.

Once you understand how viewers are being used and manipulated by shadowy third parties, hopefully everything else we discuss about the Trap will come into increasingly sharper relief. You will have context. It will be easier to comprehend the draw of online porn, the skyrocketing rates of porn addiction, the plummet from enjoying soft-core porn to craving content that borders on the criminal, as well as the overall potential psychological, mental, and social consequences.

Technology and the Trap

Remember how we discussed the free porn business model a couple chapters ago? The larger the audience and greater the demand, the more advertising money flows in to fund bigger, faster servers, smoother sites, flashier ads, improved loading speeds, and higher resolution. Porn sites can afford the best technology and top tech experts who are masters of crafting, manipulating, and altering the sites in ways most ordinary people can't fully fathom.

According to the paper, "Desire by Design: Pornography as Technology Industry," by Patrick Keilty:

> *These websites may seem like amateurish distribution services. However, they are sophisticated technology companies that employ hundreds of technical staff to design and develop interfaces, algorithms, data mining software, data analytics software, video streaming software, and database management systems.*
>
> *They are part of an innovative industry engaged in the kinds of algorithmic and data science practices that drive the profits of more widely recognized industries, such as social media, online gambling, online games, search engines, and electronic commerce.*
>
> *These designers are responsible for making strategic choices about information management and the graphical organization of content that translates into large profits, innovative capitalist media techniques, and dominant modes for curating, distributing, and regulating our experience of sexual desire today.*[5]

While the above might sound like techie word salad, we will parse out what all this means to you and all of us as we go along. Because if adult entertainers and porn viewers aren't the adversaries as we have all been traditionally led to believe, then who is the actual enemy?

Remember the invisible hand I just mentioned? That techie word salad from Patrick Keilty's paper comprises some, but not all of the parts that make up an economic system that simply could not exist before the digital age. The economic sector of surveillance capitalism powered by adult content is what I have been calling the Trap.

Surveillance capitalism asserts that human experiences are a free raw material that can be covertly mined for hidden commercial practices of extraction, prediction and ultimately sales. This business model trades in human experiences, turning them into profits without our knowledge or consent.[6]

Welcome to *The Matrix*.

You are no longer a person with free choice or free will. While the surveillance capitalist system will definitely provide us the illusion of free choice and free will, it is only because fantasy makes us a better battery.

There is a good reason many porn sites are crafted to appear amateurish. If a site looks like someone's cousin with two years of junior college threw a site together on a shoestring, then viewers let down their guard. Why wouldn't they? Who would expect a site so cluttered and seemingly disorganized to be a clever camouflage obscuring of the work of some of the most talented and brilliant computer minds of our time?

There are many ways these companies profit off our everyday experiences without us even being aware. Though the Trap employs countless tools to profit off our online behaviors, we don't need to know about or understand them all to grasp that our world is in a crisis.

If a site gathers information to improve a product, experience, or customer service, this is not what Zuboff would deem as surveillance capitalism. The reason is that the information being gathered remains in a closed system. A company is collecting data to improve a product or service.

Yet, when companies start compiling our likes, dislikes, and online actions and then view this body of raw data as a free commodity they can take then sell to unknown parties for unknown purposes, that is crossing a hard ethical line.

Gathering data isn't in and of itself the problem. When it comes to how this raw data is being used, especially in the realm of online porn, buckle up.

The Illusion of Control

Trust me, we are going to keep going deep behind the scenes, and I will explain the impact of porn's transition into cyberspace. For now, let's refer back to Keilty's list of tech employees and experts that are standard issue for any major porn site: web designers and engineers who develop interfaces, those who manage and craft algorithms, programmers writing data mining code, data analytics software, video streaming applications, and database management systems.

Picture in your mind a porn site with hundreds of technical staff. Which begs some sticky questions, such as, "Why would the porn industry funnel such vast amounts of money into collecting, storing, and sorting vast amounts of data?" More questions cascade down from just that: how is this data used when it comes to online design and experience, what is the cumulative effect of these practices on the users?

For now, I will keep it simple. It is about control. More specifically, it is about giving users a false sense of control when the system on the other side of the screen is so complex even its creators can barely keep pace with all that it does. Online porn sites use advanced software to record clicking and viewing behavior because the more information they get, the better they become at building behavioral models that can most accurately predict not only what we will do online today, but what we will likely do tomorrow, and the next day, and the next.

Once these unseen data systems collect a detailed record of what we are already doing online, third party players, such as advertisers, can then pay these puppet masters to introduce small changes that nudge our online behavior without our even being aware. For anyone who wants to know more, Silicon Valley legend Jaron Lanier expounds on this phenomenon brilliantly in his book, *Ten Arguments for Deleting Your Social Media Accounts Right Now*.[7]

But back to the topic at hand, persuasive design technology (PDT) is one of many tools that software engineers use in order to maximize the chances that we will not only engage with a site, but also remain longer and keep returning.[8] Most of us are familiar with PDT to the point that we have probably never even noticed it.

Before we go further, I want to be clear. Persuasive design technology is not, in and of itself, good or bad. Currently, PDT is embedded into all kinds of technology and sites to streamline and improve our online experiences. For instance, if a site is too hard to maneuver or requires too much work from our end, we are less inclined to stick around. If we instant message someone and see those little animated ellipses appear, there is a far greater chance we will wait for a response and keep chatting. Social media sites use PDT all the time. You might recognize this as photo tagging, alerts, waves, emojis, and auto-fills for forms. Or, say you hop onto a website, and they want you to sign up for a newsletter. The designers might add in an auto-fill function so that you don't have to type in all your information by hand.

Though elements of PDT can be used for good, recently there has been a massive outcry from psychologists, special interest groups, and software engineers and designers regarding the ethics behind the ways PDT is being deployed. This is the sticky issue with technology. Technology doesn't have a conscience; it only has objectives. There is no right or wrong, only effective or ineffective. So, when we discuss any of the technological and psychological levers brands or companies employ, we need to remember that profit is the goal, plain and simple.

Ultimately, site design is crucial when it comes to hooking viewers in the online porn world. Design and incremental tweaks increase viewer engagement which, in turn, increases demand for more content. The greater the demand, the easier it is for porn distributors to recruit new performers to willingly contribute new material. Then, the more content for audiences to explore, and the more seamless and curated the viewer experience, the better the odds that those who already watch will remain watching or even become completely absorbed. This last effect is akin to what psychologist Mihaly Csikszentmihalyi referred to as "flow."[9]

In the *Wired* article, "Go with The Flow," Csikszentmihalyi defined flow as:

Being completely involved in an activity for its own sake. The ego falls away. Time flies. Every action, movement, and thought follows inevitably from the previous one, like playing jazz. Your whole being is involved, and you're using your skills to the utmost.[10]

Flow can be wonderful. We have all experienced it. Athletes call it getting in the zone. Maybe you start drawing, painting, playing an online game, or dancing, and everything else fades out. Unfortunately, online porn sites aren't exactly wanting us in the flow as much as they want to lure us over into the dark side of flow, a state that MIT anthropologist Natasha Schüll calls "the machine zone."[11]

Schüll spent over a decade traveling to Las Vegas trying to understand the explosive profitability of slot machines since gambling entered the digital era. She wanted to understand how game designers optimized the machines to keep people playing. After talking to gamblers and casino operators about the new breed of machines, she realized that most of the people playing weren't trying to make money, as much as they craved getting into what she eventually referred to as the machine zone.[12]

One of the most predominant psychological tools porn sites embed into their coding is referred to as positive intermittent reinforcement, which is the same tactic used in slot machines. Make the colors bright and shiny, the rewards unpredictable, and it is a fairly solid formula for introducing, refining then reinforcing addictive behaviors without those on the other side even being aware they are being manipulated and herded into the machine zone.[13]

This is detailed in the July 31, 2013, article by Alexis C. Madrigal in *The Atlantic*, "The Machine Zone—This Is Where You Go When You Just Can't Stop Looking at Pictures on Facebook: What an anthropologist's examination of Vegas slot machines reveals about the hours we spend on social networks,":

What is the machine zone? It's a rhythm. It's a response to a fine-tuned feedback loop. It's a powerful space-time distortion. You hit a button. Something happens. You hit it again. Something similar, but not exactly the same thing happens. Maybe you win, maybe you don't. Repeat.

Repeat. Repeat. Repeat. Repeat. It's the pleasure of the repeat, the security of the loop.[14]

In this same article, Schüll is quoted as saying, "Everything else falls away. A sense of monetary value, time, space, even a sense of self is annihilated in the extreme form of this zone that you enter."[15]

Granted, this article is talking about slot machines and seeks to offer an explanation as to why social media can be so habit-forming. Exactly how do we end up losing hours scrolling and engaging in an activity that, if we took a step back, doesn't have a tremendous amount of real-world payoff? The people at the slot machines are chasing the same sort of high that many of us chase on social media and that viewers chase when watching online porn.

Slot machines might be mostly confined to Las Vegas, so we can dismiss that as an example that applies universally. But social media is everywhere. How many articles have we seen in the past few years that discuss the overwhelming number of apps and amount of content that constantly vie for our attention? All of that pales in comparison to the amount of porn that is available online. The sheer volume of content amplifies the chances that porn will reach more eyes, so more opportunities to serve ads to a potentially captive audience.

More ads mean more money to hire even better technical experts to refine and perfect sheepdog code that nudges and eventually herds audiences into this dark side of flow, making them chase ever greater highs. This cycle repeats over and over, and, with every evolution, this artificial brain that powers everything online grows larger, stronger, and faster.

If you feel I am being overdramatic, Yale professor and renowned statistician Edward Tufte once said, "There are only two industries that call their customers 'users': illegal drugs and software."[16]

The largest tech companies in the world have openly boasted about using psychology and employing techniques to hack human behavior in order to fuel three early prime directives: engagement, growth, and ads. Believe me when I tell you that porn sites, and those underwriting them, have the exact same goals. It's just business.

Or is it?

Playing the Odds

Part of why I mentioned Natasha Schüll's research is because much of the online porn system has been intentionally designed using virtually identical tactics employed by social media sites and casinos. Though, while I will point out the similarities between casinos and online porn, in my opinion, online porn is an enormously different and far more dangerous game.

First, there are two things you are unlikely to see inside a casino: windows or clocks. This is common sense from a behavioral modification strategy standpoint. Casinos want visitors to lose their sense of time because this increases the odds players will keep gambling and spending money. The casino's goal is to create an environment that is most conducive for coaxing gamblers into a hypnotic state that keeps them chasing a high.

The internet porn game uses similar tactics, but their purposes and end goals go far beyond selling porn services. There is the alternate, obscured agenda that is a far better money-maker. You would think that the porn viewer is ahead of the game compared to the casino gambler because online porn is free, so the house never collects cash. With free porn, viewers can keep their money because this house is busy collecting pieces of their human experience. These entities want you to not only lose time, but they have crafted a system that profits from your time. For them, your time very literally is money. Massive corporations are purchasing your life away, click-by-click. In porn, the odds don't merely favor the house, but the house always wins...always.

The moment a viewer clicks on a site, *ka-ching*! It doesn't even matter if the person only stays a few seconds. A person lands on the website, and then the advertiser pays the porn site for an impression. Not only that, but while on that site, digital noses have already sniffed out and collected information unique to you that will then be repurposed and sold back to the advertisers and their marketing agencies. Some distant third party made money off two-seconds of your life. The longer you stay, the more of your life you sell, only someone else gets the proceeds.

Seems like a stacked deck to me.

The second way that porn is like casinos is that the porn industry doesn't solely profit from addicts. Vegas, Atlantic City, cruise ship casinos and other venues enjoy a good gambling addict for sure. No one on staff is going to step in and stop grandma from putting her entire Social Security check into a slot machine coin by coin.

The truth is that Las Vegas doesn't need the guy who gambles away his house, car, retirement account, and kids' college funds to remain profitable. It's all about the numbers. Creating, and maintaining a steady stream of tourist gamblers is easier. There are far more people willing to lose twenty, fifty, or even a hundred dollars, give a rueful laugh, then walk away and hit the buffets. Multiply the tourist gambler by a few hundred thousand and that is a solid business plan. Bankrupting everyone who walks through the door? Not so much. Broke people don't have money to play blackjack, get a massage, or enjoy a steak dinner.

As we go on, we are obviously going to address porn addiction, but again, the addicts only make up a portion of what fuels this vast online porn enterprise. Companies are making colossal fortunes from those who might just take a peek once, or now and again. What I believe should concern you is that, though the internet porn industry doesn't require addicts, they very much want to create addicts.

Everything in the software design, the algorithms, and data structures are all tooled to increase the odds of addiction. This is because these sites are making the most money off the viewer's time and resulting data, which are clearly boosted with addictive behavior. Sure, maybe the sites are making decent money on the ad click-throughs for guaranteed enormous penis enhancements or cheap body spray. *But there is no physical product for sale.* The sites are selling the viewer an experience, then turning around and reselling the intel from the viewer's engagement either directly or indirectly.

One might be able to claim that casinos also would love to create addicts. The difference, however subtle, is in the business relationship. Because of the very nature of their business model, it doesn't serve a casino's interest financially to ruin every person who darkens their doors. The casino makes money directly from the consumer and so must maintain a more symbiotic than parasitic relationship with its visitors in order to survive and even thrive.

This is what Shoshana Zuboff would have probably considered a traditional capitalism model. Whenever anyone steps into a casino, they are generally at least aware there is an inherent risk, even danger. By agreeing to gamble, visitors are accepting the terms of partaking in the products and services offered. Collectively as a society, we acknowledge this risk and that it requires a degree of personal judgment and responsibility. This is why we have laws that only people over a certain age of consent are allowed to gamble. There is, however, a strong interdependence between the producer and the consumer. Put simply? The casino loses if their profit plan is all take and no give.

Online porn is a wholly different creature. Those watching porn are not the customers. Let me say that one more time: porn consumers are not the porn company's real customer. They are the host losing valuable nutrients the parasitic business model then uses to grow healthier and larger. The individual bits of data are re-fashioned into a valuable product for sale. Advertisers keep the money flowing, so those profiting want that skin-wrapped consumable we call a person spending as much time as possible watching porn. The porn sites don't care if you lose your job, your spouse, your mind, or your life because their algorithms can't care. Advanced software consumes everything you give it because that is ultimately what is for sale. That is the real product: your life.

If you are feeling nervous that the online porn industry wants to create addicts, what should really concern you is they already possess the power to create addicts and have been for a while now. This dovetails into my third point regarding the similarities between porn and gambling. Just like social media sites, the porn industry also stole the casino's psychological toolbox and then gave those mental levers upgrades unlike anything we have witnessed in human history.

There is this flawed belief that we humans can adapt to technology, just like we learned to adjust to the introduction of lightbulbs, cars, telephones, newspapers, radio, cable television, and twenty-four-hour news outlets. But this argument is flawed for a number of reasons. Namely, since around the middle of the twentieth century, computer processing power has increased roughly a trillion times. No other technology comes even close.[17]

Cars aren't a trillion times faster, and cable television isn't a trillion times more powerful. We are trying to keep pace with smart, self-evolving technology that is advancing exponentially every day. Meanwhile? The human brain hasn't changed much at all.[18]

Practices like persuasive design technology, positive intermittent reinforcement, and the persistent use of attention extraction models are light years ahead of our brains, even though our brains ironically conceived of and designed the initial programs. This is a race we can't run, let alone win, and humanity is only falling farther and farther behind.

Every time someone clicks on an online porn site, they are unknowingly sharpening the blade that will part their life experiences out for profit.

The More You Play, The More You Lose

Every time we hit a porn site, we hand them information that is then weaponized against us. Remember metadata, which is "data about data?" Why would Facebook want that hidden information embedded in people's images? It's because social media sites are information vacuums. Those images reveal a lot about the people posting. What are their hobbies and interests? Do they travel? Are they married or single? Do they have children? What is their occupation? How old are they? What makes them insecure?

Google and social media sites can legitimately claim they don't sell user's information to third parties because it's technically true. What they do sell, however, are behavioral predictive models they fashion together using the content we post and our behavior online. When companies have the ability to capture our browsing habits and history, they can then cobble that apparently unrelated information together into what John Cheney-Leppold referred to as an "algorithmic identity" in his paper, "A New Algorithmic Identity: Soft Biopolitics and the Modulation of Control,":

> *A person's algorithmic identity is dynamic, meaning it changes with every online engagement. What do we google? What captures our interest? What do we like, dislike, or share? How long do we stay on a site, watching a video, etc.? At what point do we leave (lose interest)? All of this 'behavioral surplus' is stored, analyzed, refashioned then used and resold.*
>
> *Is there a way to cross-index people with similar algorithmic identities and check if those with similar behavioral profiles also stopped clicking and scrolling at the same point? If so, what was that point? Can they change the font, the color, the ads, the layout? These companies are collating vast reservoirs of behavior patterns and then using that data to create better and better predictive models.* [19]

Once a company has solid predictive models, then its invisible hand starts to poke, prod, and nudge us toward its goals, not ours. Though the real genius of the trick is we will believe we chose that goal of our own free will.

This all reminds me of an eerie quote by Agent Smith in the movie *The Matrix*:

> *Did you know that the first Matrix was designed to be a perfect human world? Where no one suffered, where everyone would be happy. It was a disaster. No one would accept the program. Entire crops were lost. Some believed we lacked the programming language to describe your perfect world. But I believe that, as a species, human beings define their reality through suffering and misery. The perfect world was a dream that your*

primitive cerebrum kept trying to wake up from. Which is why the Matrix
was redesigned to this: the peak of your civilization.[20]

Like *The Matrix,* the illusion of free choice is essential for this new
capitalism to be effective. We believe we are watching this video or
visiting that site because we wanted to. We chose to. But it's the tiny
imperfections, such as not finding exactly what we want, that open
psychic gaps where the algorithms then can gain purchase. Once the
algorithms have a firm hold, those behind the scenes can reconfigure
our reality to their ends.

What can the software designers and engineers tweak to increase
the odds a viewer will slip into the machine zone? More importantly,
how can they design interfaces that all but ensure users slip into that
psychological state faster, remain longer and also keep returning time
and again for another hit? Every bit of data is used to enhance the
efficacy of such algorithms.

Again, referring back to Patrick Keilty's, "Desire by design:
pornography as technology industry,":

> *By data mining individuals' browsing habits, the online pornography*
> *industry uses 'algorithmic identities' to mediate sexual categories, to*
> *fetishize racial, class, and cultural difference, and to suggest content and*
> *advertisements. Importantly, each viewer's identity is always changeable,*
> *based on newly observed behaviour or the input of new metadata.*
>
> *The purpose of this adaptability is to create a capacity of suggestion.*
> *That is, to softly persuade viewers to continue searching for an imagined*
> *perfect image and to enable repetitive and recursive browsing, encouraging*
> *viewers to forgo the pleasures of the known for the pleasures of the*
> *unknown.*
>
> *Drawing on both individually generated data and aggregated data in*
> *calculating search results, these computer algorithms also track geographic*
> *locations, IP addresses, and viewer-generated tags, categories, and video*
> *titles.*[21]

In plain English? Online porn doesn't exist separately from everything else a viewer does on the internet. These sites are quietly gathering countless bits of seemingly meaningless information to play matchmaker. They know when a viewer clicks onto online porn, they might only have a short window of time to capture that person's attention. Thus, the faster the system can offer up a list of suggested content that appeals to that particular person, the greater the chances the viewer will remain on the site.

To give a simple illustration. A white middle-aged male living in Manhattan who reads *The Wall Street Journal* online, checks the stock market multiple times a day via the app on his phone, and is a platinum member of an online wine delivery service isn't going to see the same porn menu as a white twenty-two-year-old male from Houston who plays first-person shooter games with his buddies when he isn't watching videos about deer hunting, bass fishing, and car races. The site won't waste an ad for a NASCAR channel on the stockbroker, and it won't suggest a gourmet delivery service to the twenty-two-year-old.

Before any of this digital matchmaking can take place, however, the porn sites must first attract the viewer's attention.

11

THE BAIT

What lures viewers into the online porn Trap? Bait. Human biology and basic human needs are used to tempt the curious, and because it's a trap, there is no intention of letting anyone go.

I recently heard a story that really captured the essence of what I feel online porn does to those it ensnares. **Before we go any further, please know I am a die-hard animal lover. I own two cats and two dogs, one dog that is actually half-wolf, so this illustration rattled me. Try as I might, though, I couldn't find any better analogy to how porn uses human instinct against us. Therefore, I am giving you a trigger warning for depictions of animal suffering in the next few paragraphs, even though it's the very devastation that brings home the danger and distress.**

The Inuit peoples invented a highly effective way of baiting then killing wolves without the Inuit ever being actively involved in the hunt. They would sharpen a spear to a deadly point, then dip that spear over and over into fresh blood from a walrus, for example, letting each layer of blood freeze before coating it again. They would repeat this process until the spear was obscured under a thick blood popsicle, then finish it off with a warm layer that carried the tantalizing scent of fresh blood before planting the spear in the ice.

Then, the Inuit would leave and simply wait.

Wolves are carnivores; thus, it is in their nature to be attracted by the scent of blood. Detecting what appeared to be an easy treat, the wolves would home in on the smell and start licking the fresh blood. In their excitement, they would lick and lick and lick yet have no idea that, at some point, they were actually feasting on their own blood.

So caught up by their instinctive drive, the wolves licked and gnawed past the frozen layers to the sharpened point that in turn lacerated their tongues and mouths. Excited by a sudden rush of warm blood they were too crazed to realize was their own, they would lick even more feverishly. Eventually, the wolf would lose enough blood that it would finally collapse and die. The Inuit could simply check the trap at their leisure, gather up the dead wolf, butcher the carcass, then keep, trade, or sell anything valuable. They might even use the dead wolf for fresh blood to slather onto a newly sharpened spear meant to catch yet another wolf.

I know this is only an analogy, albeit a gruesomely appropriate one at that. However, I would like to point out that the Inuit never had any intention of hunting wolves to extinction. They trapped what they might be able to use, trade or sell. They thinned packs to stem overpopulation that might breed disease, weakness, and ultimately starvation. Starving wolves are dangerous wolves. Overpopulation isn't only bad for the packs, but it also seriously endangers any humans in the area.

Porn, by severe contrast, exhibits no similar respect or restraint, thus the metaphor ends here. Algorithms only seek to evolve and achieve greater efficacy at planting as many blooded stakes as possible to take down as much prey as possible. Instead of blood, however, porn uses something far more powerful.

Sex.

The Boobie-Trap

Humans are wired for sex. Physical attraction is hard-coded into the brain. Males are particularly visual, so graphic images make a fantastic lure. What is singularly cunning about online porn is that it uses what humans are wired to want as bait, then fails to mention the razor-sharp spear at its core.

I went through such great lengths to explain surveillance capitalism because the quasi-symbiotic relationship between the adult entertainment industry and the adult entertainment consumer has gone away. It's just that no one bothered mentioning that inconvenient fact to us, the public.

In the old market capitalist system that most of us grew up in, the porn industry was interested only in feeding a lot of hungry "wolves." Strip clubs, video stores, peep shows, and porn magazines were once vested in maintaining live, happy, well-fed "wolves." They lured in audiences willing to pay to feast regularly off something fresh—a new movie, a special issue of a magazine, an especially racy calendar featuring a nude celebrity, etc. The audience was the consumer who had to pay for the product.

The Trap altered this relationship when hidden forces made online porn free. Now, not only could anyone with internet access consume porn, but for the first time in history, traditional market barriers vanished. There was no longer any need for someone to go to a physical store for a physical product and be required to produce a legal ID. On top of this change, older pornographic content could suddenly be digitized and stored forever. Texas teacher Resa Woodward found this out the hard way.

Porn audiences suddenly enjoyed unlimited shelf space, unlimited shelf life, and unlimited access. The sheer volume of content that online sites could make available tipped the scales to their distinct advantage at the expense of the audience and society. This definitive shift away from brick-and-mortar, with all its zoning and NIMBY (Not in My Back Yard), and overhead, to click-and-mortar, turned customers into users forever after.

In this new digital dynamic, the porn industry makes far more off of selling "dead wolves" than feeding live ones. Not only that, but online porn, like many other online entities, has been able to operate unseen, unchecked, and unregulated.

They are able to spear bait all over the internet without any concern about whether the bait happens to catch children as well as adults. It isn't as if there are any consequences. While companies might insist they are only baiting for wolves, in this new economy, pups are fair game, too. Everything is fair game. Profit above all else is the only thing that matters.

Click Bait

If you have not watched the documentary *The Social Dilemma,* I strongly recommend it. For years, I had been aware some kind of trap existed, but it was like I had spotted an iceberg off in the distance. I had been in the adult industry long enough to sense something had fundamentally shifted, but I didn't know precisely what that something was.

I only sensed my industry had changed, and definitely not for the better. That, and the porn business wasn't simply getting worse, it was quickly turning into a hellscape. I stood helpless, watching fans get sicker, becoming more addicted. They would email me, confessing how they were falling into hopelessness and despair. But what could I do? I hated myself for being part of the problem and still struggle tremendously with guilt and shame. Yet, despite many attempts to wriggle free, I couldn't find my own way out of the Trap. If I couldn't find an exit, how could I tell these fans an exit even existed?

My only option was to dig in and figure out what was going on. Since I didn't have a time machine and couldn't go back and make different life choices, I had to make a decision. Either I could keep feeding the beast, or I could use my unique life experiences and education to make a difference.

Once I watched *The Social Dilemma* and started reading and researching, the pieces all began fitting together into a single ruinous picture. I was revealing a hidden reality much worse than I could have ever imagined. A reality behind our reality so to speak. I would just about finish brushing away one layer of misdirection only to realize there was more. Finally, I understood that what I had believed to be discrete events or phenomena weren't separate at all.

My goal to reveal this reality behind our reality is largely why I have written this book the way I have. We can't neatly untangle the performer, from the viewer, from the internet, from a globally connected world. If we only address the porn industry without taking a serious look at who is funding it and how, we are doomed. If we are going to dismantle the Trap, it's imperative we see the whole picture. Everyone can be negatively impacted, not only those who watch porn.

Without enough information, people can't make informed choices. We put warning labels on cigarettes, alcohol, cough syrup, spray paint, and glue. Every time we pick up a prescription, that bottle comes with a long printout of all the possible side-effects no matter how rare. There is a reason for all this information. Whether we choose to read and act on it or not is our choice, but the ball of responsibility is firmly now in our court. Regardless of what choice we make, knowledge offers us authentic and informed agency.

Many of us grew up accepting that computers would be the way of the future. Those of us in the older generations initially regarded the internet with suspicion, but that gradually faded away. Going online was optional, until it wasn't. In today's world, it's virtually impossible to function without using computers and technology. Everything is digital. We bank online, pay bills online, shop online, and we have steadily shifted to socializing online. Cell phones have replaced landlines, and we text instead of talking. Computers have become so interwoven into our daily lives most of us can't recall life before the web. Some generations have no concept of life without search engines, smart phones, tablets, and AI helpers like Alexa or Siri to guide the way. Why bother reading a map when there is GPS? Who owns dictionaries, encyclopedias, or thesauri when spellcheck, grammar check, and Wikipedia are so much faster and easier?

Everything comes at a cost. For decades, experts, doctors, and intellectuals insisted that children needed to be introduced to computers as early as possible. There were so many benefits! Not only did computers make learning fun, but upcoming generations had to be tech-savvy if they hoped to compete in a software-saturated world.

Though our society careened into the digital world at breakneck speed, we are only now getting a chance to observe and study the very real and damaging effects from being constantly immersed in an online world. Thus far, there are no warning labels on social media or internet browsing, but books and documentaries are now beginning to surface. I hope this book might be counted among those. Perhaps we can offer greater independence and return healthy levels of self-determination as well.

It won't be easy. Just like with social media applications, software engineers have not only figured out how to make porn highly addictive, but, as we will discuss here in a bit, what they are doing can fundamentally alter our brains. One might even go so far as to claim they are terraforming minds. I will use science and the latest research to support my claims in the upcoming chapters.

A Trail of Digital Breadcrumbs

How did we get here? I remember watching *The Matrix* and wondering how humans got from walking around living their lives to ending up sealed in a vat of goo powering a giant intelligent machine. What did they miss? More importantly, though, what have we missed?

In the early decades of computers and software, the industry revolved around selling physical products. Remember RadioShack? Consumers purchased physical goods like computers, floppy disks, drives, programs, printers, etc. As we charged headlong into the early twenty-first century, some companies like Apple were able to maintain a semblance of traditional capitalism, namely because they had a physical product to sell.

Sure, Apple bulldozed the music industry with the iPod. They simply used technology to give consumers what they wanted, which was a customized purchasing experience paired with instant gratification at an affordable price.

Instead of music lovers having to go to a music store to buy a physical CD of a whole album just to get one particular song, Apple riffed off what the free music service Napster had attempted but botched. Apple wasn't merely selling a new way of buying and playing music, they were selling an experience. An empty iPod without music was an incomplete sale without single-serving songs (also for sale) to go in it. Now, because of the endless options for customization, no two iPods were exactly alike. Plus, each iPod could change day to day, or week to week. Consumers could create playlists for different occasions and more, etc. Eventually, the iPod experience merged into the smartphone.[1]

On the surface, combining products seems like it's taking away a revenue stream for Apple. But it meets the consumer's demand for one less device and even opened and expanded new profit lines for the company. Apple profited from selling a very expensive physical product that the company then could optimize by offering songs for sale on iTunes. The iPhone has since opened up similar markets like digital books through Apple Books or digital entertainment via Apple TV. Apple has thus far bypassed surveillance capitalism for the simple reason that it had and still has physical products to sell that require digital content to be of any use.

What about search engine companies like Google? Or social media sites like Facebook, Instagram, Snapchat, etc.? Since they don't have physical products to sell and charging people to use their services would prove fatal, they have had to figure out ways to alter human behavior fundamentally. How could they change our habits like the ways we socialize, shop, learn, connect, and even distract a grumpy toddler? If the tech giants couldn't detour thousands of years of human habits in their favor, they would perish.

The Road to Hell & Good Intentions

I believe the early software and internet visionaries genuinely thought they were doing something good, and in many ways, they did. They connected people all over the world, opening access to information, uniting people with rare medical diseases, fueling political causes, etc. In their excitement about discovering a magic lamp, however, they failed to stop and ponder the downside or even the potential disaster they might unleash by rubbing the bottle and setting the genie free.

Be careful what you wish for because you just might get it.

Fueled by optimism, too many of the pioneers ignored the warning signs of darkness looming just over the horizon. Many in Silicon Valley turned a deaf ear to those who questioned the grand vision. They were too enraptured ushering humanity into an entirely new age, a world the likes of which we had never witnessed, and they had good reasons to be excited.

Amit Patel, a young Stanford graduate student with a special interest in 'data-mining,' is frequently credited with the groundbreaking insight into the significance of Google's accidental data caches. His work with these data logs persuaded him that detailed stories about each user—thoughts, feelings, interests—could be constructed from the wake of unstructured signals that trailed every online action. These data, he concluded, actually provided a 'broad sensor of human behavior' and could be put to immediate use in realizing cofounder Larry Page's dream of Search as a comprehensive artificial intelligence.[2]

This was a critical crossroad. Waste material was refashioned into continual learning and improvement. The more people engaged on the site, the more the site learned and could optimize for cleaner, faster, and more accurate searches.

Unfortunately, the thrill of creating a brand-new world with a wholly new ecosystem ran headlong into the dot com crash in April of 2000. Grand visions were all well and good, but no longer enough, not even for Google.

The young company struggled to find ways to reliably turn investor money into revenue. Though at the time, Google was widely considered the best of all the search engines, investors demanded more. For years, Google's founders steadfastly refused to bow to advertisers at the expense of users, but eventually they had little choice but to start making compromises. As the go-to search engine of choice, Google had already captured and stored user information and behavioral patterns solely to improve functionality. With enough data, Google could finally offer advertisers the holy grail they had never been able to find: certainty. Raw data originally used solely to improve the quality of search results was put to use connecting advertisers with their statistically ideal customers, and Google's AdWords was born.[3]

When Google shifted from using data to serve users toward surveilling them, they arguably opened Pandora's Box and unleashed a wholly new form of capitalism into the world...surveillance capitalism. Once Google demonstrated just how profitable information surplus could become, priorities shifted to improving data collection, sorting, sifting, shaping and selling.[4]

Designers introduced new technologies like web crawlers to scour for keywords and possibly useful information that could then be molded into a product. Google might have pioneered data extraction, but other companies—namely social media sites—followed close behind. Facebook launched the year Google went public and soon hired away Google brainpower to implement many of the practices that had made AdWords such a raging success.[5]

In their zeal to turn a profit, these companies and their designers seemingly forgot one of the fundamental rules of nature: an alien species may survive and even flourish in a new ecosystem, but it can also escape and become invasive and predatory. Some species can evolve faster than we—scientists, engineers, humans—can keep pace.

To paraphrase the infamous words of Dr. Ian Malcolm from

Jurassic Park, Silicon Valley was so preoccupied wondering if they *could*, they never stopped to think if they *should*.[6]

If gathering massive amounts of data was the road to riches, then online porn could be considered the superhighway. Not all humans are wired to consume drugs, cigarettes, or alcohol, but every human is wired for sex. It's the biological imperative that keeps us as a species from going extinct. The online porn industry hijacks our natural desires for their unnatural profits, consequences be damned.

12

THE TRIGGER

What triggers a person to look at porn? Basically, it's the same natural craving that lured the wolves to the Inuit death popsicle. Sex sells because our brains are designed not only to crave sex, but as much sex as possible, the more sex the better.

In the twenty-first century, it's easy to forget how fragile humans are. It wasn't all that long ago that infant mortality was a common reality. Even as recently as the mid-nineteenth century, close to 40 percent of babies born died before reaching the age of five.[1]

Humans are born completely helpless and remain that way for at least four-to-five years. This is why it was very common to have a lot of babies for most of our history. Couples had ten, twelve, or even fifteen children because the odds for survival were so slim.

Scientific, technological, and medical advances might have drastically lowered infant mortality, but that fact is a moot point to our brains. Our brains still are working off an operating system that is hundreds of thousands of years old, and a few decades of progress isn't going to change that any time soon.

Online porn sites are very grateful that our brains don't evolve at the same pace as technology, and like a virus taking advantage of an outdated security program, they take major advantages of our human weakness.

Super-Sized & Supernormal

If we start with the basic argument that humans crave sex and lots of it, then what happens with porn? First, porn is the junk food of sex. We are drawn to high calorie, high-sugar, high starch foods because food has only become plentiful within the last century. For tens of thousands of years, famines and death due to starvation were ever-present threats. Fast-forward to 2021. Our lizard brain—the most primitive neural structure that governs our basic needs—doesn't know that the drive-thru at McDonald's will still be there tomorrow, next week, or next month, so it says, "Eat up! Make sure we don't die!" Pornographic images are the high-calorie, candy-coated, deep-fried version of sex and reproduction. Porn hijacks our fundamental survival instincts using what Nobel Prize-winning ethologist Nikolaas Tinbergen termed *supernormal stimuli*.[2]

Tinbergen discovered that he could override instinctual behavior in a wide variety of creatures by simply offering them a larger, brighter, or more ideal version of the natural option.[3]

In one famous experiment, Tinbergen constructed cardboard female butterflies with larger and far more vibrant wings than their natural counterparts. He noted that once the male butterflies caught sight of the supernormal version, the males completely disregarded the real female butterflies, and all of them tried to mate with the imposters.[4]

Pornographic images trigger a stronger sexual response because they offer an extreme and artificial version of the natural: larger breasts, fuller lips, longer legs, smoother skin, on and on. So, Joe Normal might be idly surfing the web, checking out race cars or watching sports videos when that flashy ad appears off to the side with three ingredients almost guaranteed to trigger a click: bright colors, a supernormal sexual image, and the word *free*.

Free porn offers the supernormal bait that triggers the target audience to enter the porn site's domain, then keeps serving up more supernormal images to increase the odds their algorithms will create a captive audience. Remember, in a surveillance capitalism system, the longer a viewer remains on the site, the more valuable that person becomes. Joe Normal doesn't think he is doing any harm. In fact, he is only doing what is natural. He is watching what would interest any other guy just like him, and it's free. No one forced the people on the screen to have crazy sex. He didn't dip into the grocery budget to buy the videos. It's no harm, no foul.

What Joe Normal doesn't realize is that every moment he is on these sites, advanced software is scouring his data, monitoring his behavior, and capturing that information. The advertisers funding free porn and the porn site owners have a vested interest in nudging Joe Normal into the machine zone so that they can gather enough intel to eventually maneuver him toward or connect him to certain products and services. The longer he stays, the more time the site potentially has to nudge him closer and closer to addiction. If he stays on the site long enough, then odds are favorable that he will no longer get as much of a thrill out of the free porn and will be more receptive to the paid services.

Even if Joe Normal never escalates to the paid services, he is still valuable because it doesn't take long for the site's artificial intelligence to know him better than he knows himself. If he is a white male over forty, then forget the acne cream and body spray ads. Replace those with ads featuring a cure for premature balding, a drug that reverses erectile dysfunction, or a dating site brimming with single Asian women.

Why Asian? The software picked up on what kind of female not only attracted Joe Normal's attention but also kept his attention. If his algorithmic profile indicated he preferred blondes, redheads, college coeds, or even other men, the site would instantly reconfigure to fit his ideal, then offer him more of what he never realized he even wanted.

Over time, this subtle digital maneuvering can have terrible physical and psychological effects and can completely alter Joe Normal as a person. He might click on the free porn to watch hot blondes and rather tame porn, only to realize ten months later he can't get aroused unless he watches videos featuring extreme violence, depravity and torture. His own brain has betrayed him, turning him into a literal junkie for dopamine.

Dopamine Rush Hour

Since this chapter is about triggers, let's talk about the biggest, baddest trigger there is: the dopamine rush. Porn triggers a dopamine response that floods the body's reward system and creates a high that is designed to reinforce good behavior like eating a great meal, working out, or having fantastic sex. These are all behaviors that help us thrive and survive both individually and as a species. Dopamine is there to encourage us to keep repeating these positive, healthy actions.

The problem is that the human brain apparently can be tricked as easily as a butterfly brain. What Joe Normal sees while surfing porn is a fiction, but his brain rewards him as if he were actually having great sex. This dopamine rush is the most common gateway for a full-blown addiction.

Let's start with the fact that porn has always had an addictive component. Curiosity alone can trigger someone to click on that ad. But, as we all know, life comes with its fair share of problems. Boredom, loneliness, or some life crisis can tip a person who normally might ignore porn to giving it a glance. Financial trouble, relationship problems, depression, or grief can also prompt Joe Normal to take that initial peek into the porn world.

But what happens when supernormal crises collide with supernormal temptation? For instance, Joe Normal finds himself, like everyone else on the planet, in the middle of a global pandemic. Like any human, he is always vulnerable to veering down a path he never imagined. I think it's safe to say most of us have experienced that perfect storm of events that totally changed the game for us. Hit with hard times, even really hard times, we still found our way through, though not without bruises and scars. Then there is the supernormal crisis, the emotional sixty-car pileup that happens when life as you know it disappears down an unforeseen sinkhole. Joe Normal is obviously a fictional example, but many people in the United States actually are experiencing eerily similar circumstances, so this example isn't as extreme as it might have been a year or two ago.

What About Joe?

A month after COVID-19 hit headlines and lockdowns hit every state, Joe Normal had to close his small business and lay off all his employees. Though he vowed to all of them he would figure out a way to reopen and believed it at the time, now he is not so sure. Two weeks after closing the business, his wife was furloughed from her corporate job.

Their three kids are home and driving him bonkers, mostly because they have too many questions, and he has too few answers. Both he and his wife are struggling, uncertain, and afraid. Neither Joe nor his wife can figure out how to maneuver their three kids in three different grades into the right Zoom classes or keep an eye on them to make sure they aren't goofing off on YouTube or TikTok instead. They can't go to church together, the gym, the beach, or even a park. Now, they are all cooped up inside.

Joe Normal feels anything but normal. He feels like a total and complete failure. The house that once gave him so much pride is the same one that now he might very well lose. Whenever he looks at his wife, the woman he loves with all his heart, all he can think about is how much he has let her down. He had promised to take care of her and their children, and he has failed everyone in every way. How could he be so stupid? His dad wanted him to be a doctor, a lawyer, an accountant. Get a real job. Something safe. But he had chosen to be an entrepreneur instead, and it had worked out great. His business had given them a very nice life for almost seventeen years.

What did he fail to see, to prepare for? He knew he shouldn't have indulged his wife and kids so much with vacations and gifts, but his old man was always busy at the office and never home. What was the point of working so hard if you never enjoyed life? It felt so good to make them smile, but was he a fool? He had thought he was being a great dad, a good husband. In retrospect? He was an idiot. He is a total loser.

Every mistake, every flaw, every could have, would have, should have scrolls through his mind nonstop and there is nothing to take his mind to a better place. The news is all doom and gloom with no end in sight. Usually, Joe Normal would have gone to the gym to blow off steam, but he had to cancel their membership to save money. Not that it mattered, since the gym has been closed for the past three months anyway. He can't go to church, visit his parents in the neighboring state, or even hang out with his friends and play cards and laugh like they used to. He would be too ashamed to face them anyway. What is he supposed to tell his father? How can he look his friends in the eye? The ones who are all "essential" employees. They once looked up to him, and now that all feels like a seriously sick joke.

He used to pass the time on social media, but the relentless onslaught of angry and hopeless posts is only making him even more irritated and depressed. All he feels is despair. Joe Normal has stress upon stress heaped upon stress.

Do you think he might need a good rush of dopamine right about now?

One night, after tossing and turning far too long, Joe thinks he will do what he used to do back when the business stressed him out. He would get online and wind down reading specs on high performance cars. He slips into his office, scrolls through some articles, and then this ad pops up. They are always popping up, but he has always ignored them. Good way to get a computer virus or, if he listened to Father Murray, to go to hell. But he is already in hell, so what the hell, right?

Joe's eyes dilate, his heart races, and everything starts to tingle, and he thinks, "Why not?"

His environment, the challenges and stressors have primed him not only to click on that site, but to keep clicking. Hey, the content is free, and that is right in Joe's price range. Besides, he is a grown man. Adrenaline rockets through his veins, and his blood feels practically carbonated. He isn't just feeling good, he is practically high! In fact, he feels better than he has felt in months, maybe even years. Why had he been avoiding this stuff for so long?

Maybe there is a twinge of guilt when he thinks of his wife, but these women aren't real. He isn't cheating. In fact, he wants his wife more than he has wanted her in ages. After watching for a while, he can't take the pent-up sexual pressure anymore and heads back to the bedroom and wakes up his wife. He even throws in a couple moves he saw on one of those videos.

She is a bit shocked but seems to like it. He definitely likes it. He didn't know how much he had missed her, or at least how much he missed being a man. Joe falls off to sleep curled up with his wife and has the best rest he has had in months.

This is simply the beginning of the story, though.

There is a problem here. Joe Normal isn't the only one in this house primed with triggers. This is where the debacle of online porn becomes extremely complicated.

During the first half of this book, we explored the experience, perspectives, and predicaments adult entertainers endure. But adult entertainers are of legal and consenting age, barring illegal content from sex traffickers or predators. Now, we are stepping into a strangle-vine of epic proportions because viewers of online porn can be adults, but many are children. Joe Normal's path to potential porn addiction shares much in common with his son, yet at the same time, there are vast differences. As Joe Normal and Joe Junior tread deeper into the Trap, each phase will be markedly different psychologically, physiologically, and socially.

What About Joe Junior?

We can see that Joe Normal is having a rough time. But his son, Joe Junior, has his own troubles. Right before the shutdowns, he had just been selected as the first-string pitcher on his school's junior varsity baseball team and was well on his way to being a top candidate for college scouts by next season. Now, there is no baseball, no spring break at the beach with his friends, no spring dance, no summer vacation in Cabo. Though his parents try to hide it, he knows they're fighting non-stop about money. On top of that, his two younger siblings hog the television to play stupid little kid games. His parents make him babysit all the time, which is completely unfair. They aren't *his* kids. Why is he taking care of them?

Joe Junior has the natural urges and impulses of a hormonal fifteen-year-old boy, but he is stuck at home bored, isolated, angry, resentful, and riddled with anxiety. He can't go to the batting cage, can't play ball, and their backyard is too small even to practice his pitching, so in addition, he is worried that he will lose all the skills he has worked to build for most of his life. Will he even be good enough to play once everything reopens?

He and his new girlfriend used to text all the time. But when it got out that his dad's business closed, she didn't text as much, and then she eventually stopped responding at all. He kept asking her if something was wrong, but she just kept telling him she was busy. How could she be busy trapped at home with nothing to do? He is pretty sure she has hooked up with that senior on the varsity baseball team, the one all the girls at school want to date, at least it seems like it from social media. She likes and comments on everything he posts, down to his stupid scrambled egg whites video.

When Joe Junior shuffles off with his laptop to do his homework, he does what his buddy in Algebra II told him to do. He switches the Wi-Fi to his elderly neighbors' Wi-Fi. Joe Junior knows their password because his mom volunteered him to go over and help set up their internet. He had made their password something super simple they could remember. But guess what, he can remember it, too and they never bothered to change it. Now, he can surf the web without all the stupid parental controls that were really for his stupid little siblings anyway.

What happens when Joe Junior is on his favorite gaming site and that pop-up ad featuring two nearly nude women kissing beneath a bright bold title, "Hot Horny Stepmoms: WATCH FREE!" appears? He is only fifteen, but, when he clicks, the site just makes him check a box that makes him promise he is old enough to watch. Joe Junior hits play, and he experiences the same dopamine high and adrenaline rush as his dad.

Let's pause here, though. The son's encounter isn't entirely the same as his father's. In this scenario, we are going to make the assumption that Joe Junior is not yet sexually active. Until this new girlfriend, he has been pretty much all sports all the time and has never been in a relationship. Maybe he has enjoyed a few kisses and perhaps a fumbling slide for second base, but all that shut down with school. He is now alone while also awash in the hormones of puberty.

Thus, when the "Hot Horny Stepmoms" video plays, and he witnesses something he has never seen and only barely believed existed, dopamine and oxytocin flood his brain.[5] His male body also responds the way in which it was designed. Yet, moments after viewing what is happening on the screen—unfamiliar images, sounds, language—he also feels fear and uncertainty, stressors that trigger his body to also release cortisol.

This is a chemical cocktail of a sexually traumatic experience.

According to Seattle therapist Matt Morrissey's April 17, 2019, article, "How Early Porn Exposure Traumatizes Boys and Fuels Toxic Masculinity,":

> A boy's anatomy allows for little subtly in the realm of arousal. His sexual organs live outside of him. And despite the brain's signals of danger and fear, often his penis exposes just how alive his heart feels. His ambivalence is concretized; he is both afraid and intrigued. And often, he will begin to chase the feelings of fear and pleasure, continuing to link them in his brain. And in a toxic masculinity culture, the loop of risk-taking and pleasure-seeking is praised and expected, even if it only happens in secret.[6]

Unlike his father, Joe Junior is alone, and this life-altering incident is a secret. With no sexual partner, he masturbates for physical release. It's not that he hasn't ever masturbated before. He is a young, hormonal male. But paired with this video, the pleasure is beyond anything Joe Junior has ever known. Not long after this super rush, though, he might feel the crushing sense of shame, contempt, or even revulsion about what he just felt and did. What's more disquieting, though, is those feelings will quickly pass, and soon, Joe Junior will hardly be able to wait until he can repeat this behavior again and again.

I would like to underscore that something far larger has happened here with Joe Junior, other than treading into perilous addiction territory. This is much more than a curious teenager watching a porn video. His young brain is constantly observing the world around him, forming connections and crafting meaning from those connections. For Joe Junior, this video has fundamentally redefined the meaning and value of sex.

Ideally, sex should be grafted into other acts of intimacy with another person. Sex is a wonderful, physical demonstration of intimacy designed to strengthen a relationship with a partner. Sadly, this healthy version and concept of sex has been hijacked and rerouted. Sex no longer includes flirting, courtship, romance, longing, communication, building trust, and creating, strengthening and maintaining an emotional bond. It's no longer the fulfillment of a relationship won with work, sacrifice, and care.

Sex has now become easy and cheap, devoid of meaning. It's also now shameful instead of celebrated. These experiences are also priming him for the development of paraphilia, which, though not all of them are inherently bad, can push certain predilections to the point of becoming unhealthy, intrusive, and destructive. Sex is something to be hidden, not shared. It's an act done in isolation and solely for the self, a one-sided experience.

Why does Joe Junior need to worry what a girlfriend wants, needs, thinks, or feels when all he needs is Wi-Fi and some privacy? With easy access to online porn, Joe Junior is in for a lot of reprogramming. But, for now, he is flying high. So long as he is quiet and out of his parents' hair, they leave him alone because they have their own problems. They never suspect what he is watching because they believe they have put in safeguards to keep their kids from accessing any adult content, which they have. They didn't, however, consider their son could use someone else's Wi-Fi, and they certainly hadn't factored in the elderly neighbors who didn't change their Wi-Fi password. Kids are smart, and this is so often underestimated.

See how easily triggers can shift into a spin? Young boys are male, and males are, by and large, wired to find naked women attractive. Besides, porn is taboo, wild, and thrilling, something that is just right for an adolescent testing the limits of authority and trying to define their individual identity. It is also completely accessible to three young boys who aren't even old enough to drive. Two boys aren't even out of elementary school, but they could, in this scenario, watch all the roughest, weirdest, raunchiest videos porn has to offer so long as their parents don't catch them. Statistically speaking, Joe Junior is the most likely to show his younger siblings not only the Wi-Fi trick, but to also introduce them to something that will blow their minds.

In fact, young boys and girls, adolescents in particular, are arguably more attracted to watching porn because they are naturally curious about sex. The problem is that porn is the worst place anyone could look for sexual education. Additionally, teens could be more vulnerable to the allure of extreme porn because their brains aren't yet fully developed.

The prefrontal cortex helps control emotional impulses, assess risks, recognize danger, and appreciate long-term consequences. In adolescents, it is only beginning to develop. The amygdala, the part of the brain associated with emotions, impulses, aggression, and instinctive behavior, is then left in control. Add in porn, and this is a recipe for disaster because, as we will discuss later, pornography has been shown to alter the brain's physical structure. Adult brains have a certain amount of what is called "plasticity" as well, but adults still possess a fully developed brain. When it comes to young people, their brains are far more malleable because they are still a work in progress.

According to the July 28, 2011, article by Alexandra Katehakis, Ph.D., MFT, in *Psychology Today,* "Effects of Porn on Adolescent Boys,":

> *Between the ages of 12 and 20, the human brain undergoes a period of great neuroplasticity. The brain is in a malleable phase during which billions of new synaptic connections are made. This leaves us vulnerable to the influence of our surroundings and leads our brains to be 'wired' around the experiences and information that we receive during that time period.*[7]

All this aside, for now, my made-up example features an entire household of males, two of which are riding the dopamine rush, unaware they're possibly heading for a crash.

We all have triggers. Life will always dole out boredom, hardship, heartbreak, stress, and setbacks. What's the saying? "We are only human." When we know how those triggers work and how, if we are unwise, they can lead to major problems, we can make better choices and be vigilant when it comes to ourselves and our children.

The world of online porn promises mind-blowing experiences and endless novelty, but as things stand, this world also omits any warnings of potential dangers. These sites also shift sole responsibility for keeping minors away from their content to parents and guardians. The cigarette, alcohol, gun, and gambling industries can't get away with that, so why does online porn?

My point, as I have hopefully maintained, isn't so much to shame sex and demonize an entire industry. That would be hypocritical and unproductive. Shame and guilt are always counterproductive. We all get stressed, bored, lonely, tired, and porn promises an escape.

Just be wary of what this escape offers and the real price of entry and that children can easily gain entry as well.

13

THE DOOR

Remember those naive young people who never would have believed they would end up trapped in the adult entertainment industry's inescapable labyrinth? The Trap also uses similar half-truths and full-out lies to lure those who view porn into a similar warren of ever-shifting twists and turns and end up financially supporting and emboldening the very trap that keeps them snared. *It's no big deal. Sex is healthy and natural. No one is forcing you to watch. You can stop any time. It's harmless.* Sound familiar?

Online porn sites have a vested interest in making what they offer not only appealing, but also give the impression that it's healthy, normal, and safe. However, when it comes to their business model, online porn shares a lot in common with social media sites and search engines in that they all profit most from prolonged user engagement. By now, you know what this means. If the service is free, then you, the viewer, are the real product.

This has been the major shift when it comes to pornography. As I already mentioned, the Trap used the adult industry we had always known until it could reach a critical threshold where it no longer needed that industry to entrench and expand. The Trap doesn't make money off magazine subscriptions or video/DVD rentals and sales, and it doesn't want to. It would be absurdly unprofitable. Under the internet-based surveillance capitalism model, those behind the Trap are making more money than they ever dreamed possible. Freed from the fetters of the traditional business models—no physical products to push, warehouse space, logistics, shipping, amortization, etc.,—they have expanded the profit margin to unprecedented levels. Additionally, a web-based model permits them to operate globally where business can grow unchecked, unregulated, and largely unpoliced.

The door no longer has any real barriers to entry. All one needs is a device such as a smartphone, computer, or tablet and access to the internet. No more embarrassing encounters with a clerk, no more praying that no one you know sees your car in a parking lot at an adult establishment, no more need to present a legitimate ID, no paper trail that might reveal a porn habit. The door is shiny, wide-open, and our little secret.

It is reasonable to assume most people who click on that ad or link also believe they are in control. Adults might acknowledge porn can be addictive, but they think they will be the exception. Maybe that is true. It certainly is true for millions of adults who watch adult entertainment, just as much as it's true for millions of people who enjoy a glass of wine or a beer now and again. Just like every person who drinks a cocktail isn't automatically doomed to end up a raging alcoholic rendered homeless and living on the streets, not every person who watches porn will go down the dark paths we are going to explore throughout the rest of this book.

However, the problem is that enough viewers are going down this path that we need to wake up and take the Trap extremely seriously. So yes, many viewers hop onto the web and enjoy online porn believing they will be fine, that addiction is only for lesser, weaker people. But remember, every person caught in the grip of any serious addiction once believed the same thing.

When it comes to young people watching porn, the stakes are much higher. There are sound reasons why we don't let ten-year-olds drive cars, carry guns, buy cigarettes, or drink alcohol. As a society, we appreciate how delicate and irrational young minds are and why we need to keep them away from certain substances, activities, and content until they are older, gain maturity, and are able to make better decisions.

We wouldn't let a thirteen-year-old gamble at a casino, drink at a bar, buy a stack of lottery tickets, or even purchase a bottle of cough syrup. Yet, so long as that same thirteen-year-old checks a box "promising" he is over eighteen, the porn door is unguarded and unlocked, and he can watch all the free porn he wants.

Certainly, no one clicking that free porn link actually appreciates they have just stepped into the path of a real and present danger. Young kids definitely don't. The Trap benefits when viewers step through the door they don't even see. Or, if they do, they don't happen to notice there is no doorknob on the inside. Once the prey steps through, biology will step in and seal the deal.

The trigger is whatever leads to that first click on the bait—the ad or even a word-of-mouth curiosity to go to a site directly—that opens and entices the viewer through the door where they get that first hit of dopamine. That dopamine high feels so amazing, the viewer wants more. If dopamine were the only part of the equation, that alone could be enough to spark an addiction. The problem is that recent research demonstrates that our brain's reward center is actually made up of two different neural systems, one for "liking" and another for "wanting."[1]

Let's follow Joe Normal and Joe Junior to see how this plays out.

The "Liking System"

The liking system is a smaller part of the brain, responsible for doling out rewards for good behavior.[2] It lit up when Joe Normal met his wife, when he had his first son, Joe Junior, when he finally turned his first profit with his small business, or even when he cheered his favorite football team during the Super Bowl, surrounded by good friends.

The liking system lit up for Joe Junior whenever he hit that grand slam, aced his final exams, or held hands with his first girlfriend.

The problem is that this part of the brain lights up for counterfeit rewards, too. It doesn't matter if we are talking about Joe Normal or his teenage son, Joe Junior. Cigarettes, drugs, alcohol, and yes, porn, all trigger the same feel-good rush.

The human brain, as we discussed, releases a dopamine high for survival reasons.[3] Yet, the brain knows that this reward system also needs a counterbalance if we ever hope to function normally. Right as we experience the high pumped out from the reward centers, our brain then also goes to work producing CREB, a chemical responsible for pumping the brakes, so to speak.[4] CREB is there to help taper down that initial high and return us back to a normal state. It generates a sense of contentment and satisfaction which then allows us to return to everyday life. CREB is a critical part of our brain chemistry because it would be impossible for us to function if we were perpetually in a hyper-aroused state.

Herein lies the problem, though. Whenever a person engages in a behavior, consumes a substance, or participates in any pleasurable activity in excess, the levels of CREB start building up in the brain. As CREB levels increase, whatever once gave us that intense high, over time, starts to have less and less of an effect until it can eventually deaden altogether.[5]

Research indicates that it's this buildup of CREB that creates tolerance, which can fuel addiction.[6] We see this all the time with long-time addicts. The amount of cocaine a long-term coke addict requires to simply feel a small jolt would probably kill a first-time user.

According to the article, "Why Consuming Porn is an Escalating Behavior,":

Some researchers believe that an excess of CREB is the reason addicts experience tolerance, which means that they feel less enjoyment from the stimulant and need to use more of it to reach a high. In fact, too much

CREB floating around in your brain can dull the enjoyment of anything,
which may be why addicts often feel bored, detached, and depressed. [7]

The "Wanting System"

The wanting system takes up a lot more reward center real estate when compared to the liking center. When the brain experiences intense pleasure, this center prompts the brain to rewire new connections. Using a protein known as DeltaFosB,[8] the brain creates new neurological pathways to make it easier for the person to remember and be able to repeat this positive experience.

Keep in mind, however, that there is a good reason this area of the brain is referred to as the wanting system. Those fresh neurological connections are behind the craving to repeat that original pleasurable experience. This is where things get dicey, though. The craving propels us to repeat a certain pleasurable experience. Repetition, over time, makes those nerve connections increasingly stronger and the craving more intense. Cravings grow more powerful, which, in turn, drive us to repeat the behavior yet again. This cycle is what eventually can become a full-blown addiction.[9]

But the story doesn't stop here. DeltaFosB will also connect environmental and sensory details and associate them with the experience. Researchers call these "cues."[10] For instance, if someone is an alcoholic and a smoker, that person might not only have to stop drinking alcohol but also stop smoking to successfully kick the addiction.

Why?

Because lighting up a cigarette and even the smell of cigarette smoke are common triggers or cues to also have a drink. Since cues can be almost anything the brain has selected to connect to the experience, an alcoholic might need to change friends, avoid certain restaurants, or avoid old hobbies like watching sports if watching sports was always paired with drinking.

Porn isn't exempt from this process. DeltaFosB can turn anything into a trigger that sparks the craving to watch porn. It can be a certain time of day, a smell, a common stressor, having alone time, or literally anything at all. The pathways become steadily more sensitized the more the person watches porn until their entire world seems to be nothing but a collection of cues screaming that it's time to hop online.

This is where we get to the one-two neurological sucker punch of porn. The more someone watches porn, the more sensitive the Wanting system becomes, because DeltaFosB is fashioning cues out of everything, making the cravings stronger. Simultaneously, the liking system has been dumping CREB into the brain, dulling and even deadening any pleasurable feelings.

Speaking plainly, the result is that the person wants more and more of something that gives him less and less pleasure, porn included.

FREE Porn Door

Though we have just gone over some basic brain science of addiction, most who have just stepped through the door are in that honeymoon phase where the brain is happy to dole out rewards.

An Emory University study of behavioral neuroscience clearly demonstrated that the amygdala, the emotion control center of the brain, showed significantly higher levels of activation in males viewing sexual visual stimuli than in females viewing the same images.[11]

In English? Sexual images elicit far higher levels of arousal in men than they do in women. This in turn means men are more susceptible to the lure of online porn and thus more likely to step through the door. Does this mean that women aren't vulnerable to the siren's song of porn? Of course not. This simply means that, statistically speaking, most porn entertainers are female, while most porn viewers are male.

Females do watch porn, but usually for different reasons. Yes, good old-fashioned curiosity is enough to prompt girls to watch porn, and some do it for masturbatory pleasure, but more often than not, women watch porn to please their partner. I could write an entire book on females and porn addiction. Women aren't immune, but we are different enough that this topic merits a lot more time than I can dedicate here beyond warning that, yes—girls and women—we can fall into this side of the Trap, too.

If a female's partner is already trapped in the addiction cycle of porn, she is more likely to watch porn to please the other party. She is encouraged to do this by magazines and experts regularly recommending porn to spice up a flagging sex life, despite mounting data demonstrating that porn damages relationships and families.[12] Women also might sense their partner is more distant, cold or removed and thus look to porn to see what they are missing, to see why they are no longer enough.

This happened with my first husband. I kept asking myself what was wrong with me? This is what prompted me to have my first breast augmentation. Maybe if I had larger breasts, if I looked more like the women in the magazines that captivated him, then he would want and love me. It wasn't the case for me and my ex-husband, and it's rarely, if ever, the case for anyone else trying to please a porn addict because there are deeper, darker forces at work that no partner can compete with.

Per the article, "How Porn Hurts a Consumer's Partner,":

> *Two of the most respected pornography researchers, Jennings Bryant and Dolf Zillman at the University of Alabama, studied the effects of porn and media for more than 30 years. They found that consuming pornography makes many individuals less satisfied with their own partners' physical appearance, sexual performance, sexual curiosity, and affection. They also found that, over time, many porn users grow more callous toward females in general, less likely to value monogamy and marriage, and more likely to develop distorted perceptions of sexuality.*[13]

No matter what I did, I couldn't win because I was always competing with an illusion. As my then-husband's addiction was escalating, he was craving more extreme body types, a higher and higher level of perfection that no regular person could ever meet or compete with, not long-term anyway. I could have breast augmentation, get the hair extensions, the lashes, the nails, and work out all the time, and it wouldn't have been enough because I couldn't be airbrushed in life.

Mere mortals can't compete with a fantasy, not only in appearance, but also in our actions. Porn also reduces intimacy to its most base component, the sex act. Then it twists it and keeps twisting it. The relationship that might have initially heated up, steadily grows colder because the porn-addicted party will eventually stop bonding with their partner and shift, instead, to bonding with the images on the screen. The screen offers every variety of partner, as well as limitless novelty. It's like an endless buffet of anything one might wish for. No intimate partner can be everything, can offer an infinite sea of options and choices. They are trapped in a situation where they will never be enough.

Men are more vulnerable to the door by virtue of being susceptible to visual sexual stimulation, but this is only one part of a complex problem. As I have mentioned before, our culture sanctions and almost encourages young males indulging in adult entertainment as natural recreation and rite-of passage as soon as they hit puberty. Referring back to Seattle-based therapist Matt Morrissey's article:

> *A child is not meant to participate in sexual acts. We have laws against that. And yet, the very nature of the exposure to pornography requires a boy to join in with the actors on the screen. He's required to be sexual in a way that he had never known before. And while often this happens accidentally in isolation, it is far more likely for this to occur through the introduction of a more sophisticated and mature peer or adolescent, and even in some cases, an adult. He is required to participate twofold: both with the images on the screen and with the persons providing the access.*[14]

Culturally, I feel we are unwittingly sanctioning a form of child abuse. Our society might want to write this off as, "Boys will be boys," but when so many of our young males' first sexual encounter is forced upon them by an older peer, this is child abuse.

Maybe I sound too harsh, but hear me out. I believe there is an unwritten social contract that children should be able to trust older or adult peers to shield them from harm. When an older peer or adult introduces a child to pornography, this contract is violated, but there is little to no outcry. In today's society, we wouldn't defend an adult or even a teenager who got a younger kid drunk, taught him to smoke, or got them high. When it comes to porn, though, it is as if all the rules change, and the exposure suddenly becomes okay.

This behavior feeds toxic masculinity and reinforces the double standard that favors males. If you ever glance at the comments on porn videos, most of the disgust and ridicule is directed at the females. They are sluts, whores, and viewers cheer on the males while unloading repulsion on the women, especially in rape scenarios. Even when we aren't talking about the double standard in porn, it's everywhere. For instance, a man who is sexually active is revered, while a woman would be shamed. It's far more socially acceptable for a college fraternity guy to venture out to watch exotic dancers with all his brothers as a part of male bonding than it is for a struggling female student from the same university to pay for school stripping.

We will analyze this phenomenon in greater depth as we go on, because the adult industry has always fanned the flames of objectification, dehumanization, and outright misogyny and it's only getting worse.

Ports of Entry

For now, let's go back to Joe Normal and Joe Junior. Both have been lured to step through the door using basic biology, but why and for what ends? What do the online porn sites gain from two drastically different demographics?

Joe Normal is a middle-aged man and Joe Junior is a teenage boy. Both have secretly clicked on an ad for free porn, but how did their points of entry differ?

Location, location, location. Virtually.

Joe Normal stumbled across his ad while reading about cars, whereas Joe Junior's bait floated up on a gaming site. Now, it isn't unreasonable to assume that a fifteen-year-old would read articles about the detailed specs of high-performance cars. It stretches credulity, however, for us to believe a porn ad placed on a gaming site was only meant for adult eyes. The fact that there aren't any strict regulations to keep these ads away from younger audiences is one of many grievances I have with online porn. The notion that simply promising to be eighteen is enough would be laughable if the situation weren't so dire. And remember that when the porn is free, the viewers are the raw material to create a product—the behavioral predictive models that are so valuable to advertisers. The online porn companies are not only allowed to hide behind that flimsy, "Promise you are legally old enough," nonsense, but anyone of any age who accesses their sites are considered fair game to strip-mine for profit.

Joe Junior's laptop is just as much of a gold mine of data as his father's. The algorithms are collecting and collating all that raw data that they then cobble into an algorithmic identity to ensure the right ads cross Joe Junior's screen. Junior might get the acne cream, free games, and social media ads, while his father likely will see the ads for high-blood pressure meds and weight loss pills to get rid of that middle-aged gut. Even if Joe Normal or Joe Junior never act on any of the product ads they see while surfing porn, they are still being mined for valuable raw material for the profit of others by simply watching. Remember, so long as that porn site is open and active, prying eyes are gathering other behavioral data from their social media activity to what other sorts of websites the viewer frequents.

Certainty is something marketers have longed for since the invention of sales. Every moment Joe Normal and Joe Junior participate on porn sites, they are handing away intelligence that can be sold to third parties they will never know about.

The High Cost of Free

It already bothers me that these companies are using adults. How many people watching online porn are fully aware how much of their lives and information they are giving away? Maybe the adults watching wouldn't care, but shouldn't they at least know how their behavioral patterns are being collected, collated, refashioned, and sold?

How can a person be expected to make the best choice for himself when much of the information is blurred, jumbled, misleading, or even completely hidden? The notion of consenting or non-consenting is moot here since surveillance capitalism's ultimate objective is to take advantage of how the human brain works and harness it for their goals. With the right algorithms and programs, it's astonishingly simple to mold a viewer's thinking, tastes, and preferences in a way that serves profit over people.

As we will see, online porn is designed to be addictive and to keep even adults clicking. Hidden operators will tweak the system if it senses a lull in activity. This persistent nudging over time impacts the structure of the brain. Even though adults have a fully formed brain, our brains have what is called plasticity, meaning they can be remolded and reformed. We have already talked a little about this with the war between the wanting and liking systems. Yet, that is only a small slice of how porn can rewire our thinking, habits, desires, and beliefs.

As for children and adolescents, Joe Junior's brain isn't yet fully developed. His brain reward systems are far more receptive to input, and the wrong kind of input can lead to abnormal changes in brain structure. Psychologically speaking, Joe Junior is in formative years where he is hyper-impressionable. His self-esteem, his sexuality, his views and opinions about females, sex, relationships, and intimacy are particularly vulnerable to manipulation. He is in a critical stage of development where he will start individuating, moving away from the child and forming his own self-identity. The more time he spends watching porn, the more what he believes is real and normal will shift. This reality distortion, compounded with a budding porn addiction, can have a disastrous impact on how he thinks as he forges ahead into adulthood.

It could also be reasonably argued that, unlike his father, Joe Junior is even more susceptible to the Trap's allure and negative influences since Joe Junior grew up in the digital age. Also, unlike his father, Joe Junior has no real-world experiences with intimacy, relationships, or actual sex to use as a basis for comparison. His father grew up before the internet and social media when teens went steady, attended dances, dated, broke up, made up again, and could only socialize over the phone or in person. Joe Junior has never been part of that world. Joe Normal obviously dated long enough to propose, marry, and have three children, so Dad at least has a touchstone of reality. Joe Junior has no such touchstone. The virtual world has comprised much more of what has been real for him for most of his life. The reality distortion that comes part and parcel with the digital world, could place him at an automatic disadvantage when it comes to the appeal of online porn and the games it can play with his mind.

Online porn operates much the same way as the online games or social media sites Joe Junior has been engaging with since middle school, or perhaps even earlier. The same intermittent reinforcement that kept Joe Junior entertained with games on his mom's smartphone while she was busy shopping is the same intermittent reinforcement that kept him refreshing his social feeds, and it is the same intermittent reinforcement that online porn can use to coerce him further through the door then make sure he stays once he is in.

The same persuasive design technology used to hook Joe Junior to binge on the latest social media craze is the same PDT deployed to make surfing online porn so seamless that he will slip into the same machine zone so coveted by social sites, casinos and online gambling outlets.

Groomed for Porn?

I mention all of this because the door is tempting enough all on its own. In the case of young people like Joe Junior, the vast majority of our modern youth are uniquely malleable because they have been indoctrinated to respond to the various growth hacking techniques from an early age.

What do I mean? The door is not only more tempting to upcoming generations, but young minds have been primed to be more easily and artfully manipulated and molded by the Trap's invisible hand. The Trap's aim isn't to nurture behaviors that maximize mental health and well-being. Its aim is to train behaviors that yield the highest profits, even when those behaviors are toxic. Remember, technology doesn't have a conscience, only objectives.

Young people lack the technophobia that plagues older generations who still reserve a degree of mistrust when it comes to computers. They are far more reliant on technology, more trusting, and this has shaped our young people differently than any generation before them.

According to an article by Rachel Ehmke posted by The Child Mind Institute, "How Using Social Media Affects Teenagers,":

> Teens are masters at keeping themselves occupied in the hours after school until way past bedtime. When they're not doing their homework (and when they are) they're online and on their phones, texting, sharing, trolling, scrolling, you name it. Of course before everyone had an Instagram account teens kept themselves busy, too, but they were more likely to do their chatting on the phone, or in person when hanging out at the mall. It may have looked like a lot of aimless hanging around, but what they were doing was experimenting, trying out skills, and succeeding and failing in tons of tiny real-time interactions that kids today are missing out on. For one thing, modern teens are learning to do most of their communication while looking at a screen, not another person.
>
> 'As a species we are very highly attuned to reading social cues,' says Dr. Catherine Steiner-Adair, a clinical psychologist and author of The Big

Disconnect. 'There's no question kids are missing out on very critical social skills. In a way, texting and online communicating—it's not like it creates a nonverbal learning disability, but it puts everybody in a nonverbal disabled context, where body language, facial expression, and even the smallest kinds of vocal reactions are rendered invisible.'[15]

Studies are reporting that the modern youth aren't getting driver's licenses or going on dates, and they are more insecure than any other generation. They struggle to have authentic friendships and romantic relationships. Social media has programmed an entire generation to self-soothe with technology and to distract themselves instead of learning how to confront and cope with the uncomfortable.

Why do I mention social media sites when it comes to Joe Junior? It's because these technology products were designed using psychological levers that best stimulated then steered behavior for the sole goal to maximize engagement. Period.

Child psychologists didn't design these interfaces. Pediatric neurologists didn't write the programs that recommended new content. Software engineers might have expertly coded psychological hacks into the design, but at the end of the day, they were engineers with a goal of making the most profit, not creating ethical interfaces. To be fair, it isn't until recently anyone realized the interfaces might have been harmful in the first place.

Chamath Palihapitiya, Facebook's former Vice President of Growth, when talking about the emergent years of Facebook, openly admitted in the hit documentary, *The Social Dilemma*, "So we want to figure out how to psychologically manipulate you as fast as possible and then give you back that dopamine hit. We did that brilliantly at Facebook, Instagram has done it, WhatsApp, Snapchat has done it, Twitter has done it."[16]

In the documentary, Palihapitiya is clearly remorseful. It is easy to see his early enthusiasm and contrast it with his modern regret. Hindsight is, as they say, 20/20.

We are almost two decades into this new age and seeing the changes. Feeling lonely, bored, stressed, anxious, depressed, insecure? Grab your smartphone or tablet. Hop on a gaming system. Watch YouTube. Post some selfies. While this is a fantastic business model and great news for those who profit from people addicted to their social feeds, it isn't necessarily healthy for the consumers long-term. As the old saying goes, "You are what you eat." Notice how every one of these sites offer a never-ending "feed." What happens when the feed is toxic?

We have entire generations that have grown up believing instant gratification is the norm, who have become content to substitute the virtual for the real. Sadly, though, despite having the world at the click of a button, young people are reporting record rates of anxiety and depression, and these afflictions are emerging at far earlier ages.

This sharp increase in psychological afflictions since the emergence of social media obviously can't be blamed on any one aspect of the digital age. But take a moment to think how challenging it can be to maneuver the complexity of in-person relationships. For those of us who grew up before everything was online, even we struggle with intimate partners, friends, family, coworkers, etc. Now, imagine how terrifying it would be trying to navigate the same complexities without ever fully developing a basic human survival skill: the ability to read and interpret non-verbal communication. In a sense, many young people are trying to make their way through a complicated labyrinth of interpersonal connections after being rendered interpersonally blind.

If you run any quick internet search, you will see that most experts agree that roughly 93 percent of communication is non-verbal. Body language, facial expression, and eye contact, etc., are all essential factors in deciphering the whole message. Tone of voice is another major component of communication. Anyone who has ever heard the words "I'm fine," can attest that this one word can have a wide range of meanings from, "no big deal,"-to-"I'm mad enough to stab you with a grapefruit spoon right now." When interacting online through emails, messaging, text messages or comments, we lose both the body language as well as tone of voice. This obviously leads to a tremendous amount of confusion, miscommunication, uncertainty and anxiety. To be clear, I am not claiming modern kids have no interpersonal interactions. Of course they do. But we are designed as a species to need a hell of a lot of repetitive exposure to a wide variety of interpersonal interactions in order to master even the most basic understanding of others. We need far more face time than FaceTime to develop our social skills.

With all this in mind, is it any wonder that online porn might hold even more appeal to the digital age generations? On top of this, social media, gaming, online shopping, and downloadable content have all helped groom countless young people to crave the dopamine hit as well as expect instant gratification. Having online friends and online relationships trains young minds to psychologically distance from others. Authentic intimacy then ranges from anxiously uncomfortable to frighteningly alien.

When there is a screen between us and others, we can curate our experiences on our own terms. Instead of working through arguments or hurt feelings, we simply unfollow, unfriend, or block. Unlike the old days where humans had to exert effort to make friends and create relationships, then nurture them and sustain them through good times and bad, the modern era is defined by the path of least resistance.

Relationships easily won are easily cast aside. Friends are disposable and easily replaced. Same in love. The moment the thrills and chills run their course in an online romance, and the harder parts of being in partnership become too much work, we always have the option of ghosting the other party in favor of the new relationship that has the thrills and chills. Then it's all repeat, repeat, repeat until everything feels empty and meaningless because it is.

When we add in the fact that humans are biologically wired to be social creatures, wired to have sex, I don't believe it is too big of a stretch to assert that our digital world has groomed young people to be uniquely susceptible to porn addiction. Joe Junior is far more open to the psychological levers utilized by online porn sites for the simple reason that he has been optimized to respond to them his entire life.

There are billions of doors all over the Web, most of them

unguarded, unlocked, and all surrounded with glittery ads beckoning entry. You might now be wondering just how many kids are stumbling onto porn, other than the obvious answer of too many.

Per the article, "One in 10 Visitors to Hardcore Porn Sites Is Under 10 Years Old, Study Shows,":

> *According to research by security technology company Bitdefender, kids under the age of 10 now account for 22% of online porn consumption among the under 18 age while 10-14 year-olds make up 36% of minor consumers. Internal intelligence from Bitdefender's parental control feature revealed that the under-10 age group is now accounting for one in 10 of the visitors to porn video sites. Even more unsettling, the sites most visited by children under 10 include porn mega sites which feature categories such as 'extreme brutal gang bang,' 'sleep assault,' 'domestic discipline,' and 'crying in pain.'*[17]

Unlike his father, Joe Junior is accustomed to the amorphous virtual experience. Virtual reality is reality, and that will be acutely problematic once online porn becomes part of his everyday experience.

Or should I say, if porn becomes part of his everyday experience.

The material I'm presenting might seem overwhelming, even dismal, but I am also offering hope. We can't fight what we don't see, what we might not even realize exists. We must always remember we still have power. Now that research is showing us the very real damaging effects of too much technology on children, youths, and even adults, we can choose to take control. We take control when we remove the blinders and see the web with open and honest eyes.

Those behind the Trap go to great lengths to make what it offers appear harmless for the simple reason that business thrives when we, the public, leave it alone to do as it wants. If we understand that technology has just as much potential for bad as for good, we can be mindful of how we use it. We can decide to be the driver, not just a passenger willing to go wherever the internet takes us, and we can teach our kids to do the same. Then, we are in command.

Technology itself hasn't necessarily been developed to take us any place good or bad. Technology doesn't have a conscience, as I have said. It is people programming technology to take us where it's most profitable: the Trap.

In modern life, it's common for us all to get wrapped up in our own individual worlds. I have seen it in my own house. It's a constant battle: my son playing video games online with his friends, while I am texting a friend, and my husband is bingeing the news on YouTube, and we are present, but not together. This is an easy habit much of our culture has fallen into, but what is easy isn't always what is best.

We still have the ability to shut off the phones, talk to our kids, spend quality time with our loved ones, be vigilant online, and do the extra work required for emotional and psychological health and balance. When we do this, we make it harder for the Trap to have its way with us, our children, and those we care about. Like the cigarettes, alcohol, prescriptions, spray paint, etc., we can acknowledge this product can do damage and treat it with caution and care.

Back to the Joe Normal's family...

What About Dad?

Because of his physical brain age and life experience, Joe Normal might not be initially as vulnerable as his son, but he still is susceptible to the same psychological programming. He panics when he can't find his cell phone, compulsively checks his email, glances at his screen every time it chirps with an incoming notification and has been known to surf the web while sitting on the toilet. These days, who hasn't?

Years of using computers and a smartphone have altered his behavior, routines, priorities, relationships, and even his brain structure. The liking and wanting system can wreak havoc on an adult's neurological wiring, too. But email and social media were nothing compared to what he is about to encounter with online porn.

Joe Normal has clicked that free porn ad and stepped through the door, and it's a rush. The videos distract him from the fact that his life, his finances, his marriage, and his family are falling apart. They keep his mind off his looming fears of inadequacy. In fact, these videos distract him way better than those car sites he used to go to. Porn takes the edge off all his problems. He can lock himself in his office whenever he is too overwhelmed or depressed and can click over to watch some videos. Here is the twist, though: when he first started watching porn, he was having sex with his wife to feel the release. Amazing sex, actually.

But, since he is needing to watch more frequently, this is causing some problems. In the middle of the day, when he is super stressed and he needs that thrill, his wife is otherwise occupied, perhaps working a part-time retail job to help make ends meet or tending the house and kids.

He still has sex with his wife, but he is also realizing he can get a quick fix during the day if he masturbates alone. No weird questions from his spouse, no sneaking her away from the kids for some time in the bedroom. That, and, in all honesty, having sex with his wife takes a lot more time than the few minutes he needs online to take the edge off. He never even has to leave the office and can get right back to work. A trip to his favorite porn site is much more efficient.

Which is one of the main reasons it is also so incredibly dangerous.

14

THE LOCK

I have already introduced you to the concept of the lock earlier. Frankly, there are so many types of locks, I couldn't possibly list all of them, and it really isn't necessary. Every viewer is unique, and their situation is as individual as they are. Though I don't have the time, ability, or imagination to detail every lock, I will address a handful of the most common.

The Feel-Good Lock

We have already discussed the feel-good lock. The viewer sees erotic images and experiences that dopamine rush, and, from that point on, he chases after that original high again and again.

The feel-good lock is as old as the human brain and sex, and it isn't going anywhere. It is the simplest of the locks because it is part of our biology. Every culture and civilization have had their own battles with pornography, prostitution, adultery, sexual perversion and depravity that all began with this simplest of locks. Every bordello, brothel, house of flowers and pleasure palace has relied on enticing patrons to follow the sensual instead of sense.

The feel-good lock is what turned first-timers into repeat

customers after the trigger prompted a client or customer to step through the door. The better the lock, the better the business. This lock was always powerful, strong enough to be addressed in every major religion and pervasive enough to become the center of myth and legend. Read Greek mythology and you will soon realize most of the problems were created simply because Zeus couldn't keep it in his pants.

Though the feel-good lock has always existed, it was also limited. Laws, society, and the chances of being shunned, expelled or disgraced put limits on this lock for centuries. Then, starting around the mid-nineteenth century, production alone limited pornographic content. It took time to take photographs, print naughty playing cards, make movies, create calendars, etc. Then there was another limitation: space. No store could stock every pornographic film or image ever created.

The transition of porn to an online warehouse makes the feel-good lock more potent than ever because the web has limitless shelves, nothing is ever out of stock, and there is no longer even any need to even go anywhere. Best of all, everything can remain secret.

The feel-good lock actually powers most of the internet, so we are almost blind to it. We upload post-workout pictures or a photo of our new outfit onto Instagram because we enjoy and even crave praise in the form of comments, likes, and emojis. It's easy to get lost watching YouTube or playing a video game because the feel-good lock is very adept at keeping us in the machine zone.

We are so addicted to the feel-good lock, many people can't bear to stop checking their social media accounts, even when everyone is ticked off and arguing. But stimulation is stimulation, even when it is negative. We get fidgety when we are offline, worried we will miss out on something important. This sensation has even been given a name: "FOMO," which stands for "Fear of Missing Out."

Since we are already primed for the feel-good lock in so many other areas of our lives, we are unlikely to pay it much heed when it comes to online porn, at least initially, and go so far as to think it's no big deal.

The Trap, however, has supercharged the feel-good lock into something more powerful than anything our species has ever encountered because it is free, and it is everywhere all the time. Humans' reward systems are programmed to seek plenty, and hoard against scarcity. With endless free porn, our brain pulls out a disco ball and pops the champagne to celebrate finding a resource that finally isn't scarce!

We don't need to even get out of bed to find it, unless we misplaced our phone.

That dopamine rush a person feels when first watching online porn lures them through the door. This is how, over time, the feel-good bait starts morphing into the feel-good lock. The viewer logs on to watch the same videos that gave them such a rush, but soon, there is a problem. The liking and wanting centers start warring with one another. The more a viewer watches porn, the more he craves it (DeltaFosB), but the less thrilling it becomes (CREB).

Like any other addictive substance, the user needs something stronger to get the same high. This means Joe Normal and Joe Junior might very well have started out watching relatively tame porn. Yet, once father and son begin to watch porn regularly, they are already on their way toward overtaxing their brains' reward systems and altering their brains' structures.

The Wired Lock

DeltaFosB is responsible for wiring the brain and creating fresh neurological pathways. This is a good thing if we are talking about a healthy activity.

For instance, say we are learning to play the piano. How would we start? We might begin by learning to read music, how those symbols on a page relate to where we place then move our fingers on the keys. To play music on the piano, we must then learn where to put our fingers to make certain sounds. At first, this can feel and probably does sound like torture. But, if we are passionate about learning to play piano, our reward centers are designed to give us a rush as a pat on the back for practicing. Better still, the more we practice, the more DeltaFosB goes to work, rewiring our brains and making it easier for us to place our fingers in the correct positions and to make the right combinations at the right moment. Over time, it becomes easier and easier to play the chords until eventually we don't even consciously think about it at all. Our fingers simply go where they need to go to play a certain piece of music on the piano.

How does DeltaFosB do this? As we are learning the chords on the piano, our brain first must make sense of what to do and then send the orders to our hands and fingers. As that signal zips from neuron to neuron in our heads, it activates these nerve cells to wire together into connections that eventually form what is called a neuronal pathway. You might have heard the saying, "Practice makes perfect." Well, there is another saying when it comes to brain science, "Neurons that fire together, wire together."[1]

This is the same process for playing a sport, becoming proficient at cooking, studying a language, or just about anything that requires learning. Most activities we do almost automatically all started out as cumbersome and ugly. But, over time, these actions became practically effortless. Some we can do without actually being consciously aware of what we are doing. How many times have you driven to the store and, once there, had no memory of the actual trip? This is why we need to pay attention when walking, riding a bike, or driving.

This is DeltaFosB at work. DeltaFosB carves those pathways, widens them, and makes them stronger so our brains can be more efficient, and nature just adores efficiency as a survival attribute. Can you imagine how hard life would be if we had to think through every activity we do regularly? Just think about how exhausting it would be if every time we tried to drive a car, it was always like our first time behind the wheel? What about if every time we tried to read, we had to sound out every word as if we were back in elementary school? Imagine the endless scraped knees if every time we hopped on a bicycle it was like day one without training wheels. Without these neurological pathways that make so many activities second-nature or rote, it would be almost impossible to function. We would hardly be able to learn anything, let alone retain or improve on anything we did learn. DeltaFosB plays a critical role in brain development.

Here is the catch with porn, and with porn, trust me, there is always a catch.

In chapter 10, I introduced the concept of what psychologist Mihaly Csikszentmihalyi referred to as flow. Flow is a state of hyper focus, where everything else falls away. Flow is also the most ideal environment for fashioning super strong neurological connections or wiring the brain.[2]

Now imagine Joe Normal who is awake at one o'clock in the morning watching porn. He is so absorbed in clicking from video to video that he only realizes how long he has been online when his wife knocks on the door to see if he wants any breakfast. Joe Normal has just spent anywhere from four-to-five hours deeply immersed in the most ideal mental state required for forming and strengthening neurological connections.

Joe Junior used to know a lot about flow, or as he called it, "Getting in the zone." He did this with baseball, when he practiced in the batting cage or worked on his pitching skills. But, since that activity has been replaced with sliding off quietly to watch porn, he is replacing those hours that once made him a top-notch baseball player with watching porn.

Our brain might be a small organ, but it has a monstrous appetite. Though the brain makes up only two percent of our body weight, it consumes about twenty percent of our total energy and oxygen.[3] This means there are only so many resources to go around so the neurological pathways we don't use, we lose. Any parent who has tried to help their child with geometry after decades of not using this skill appreciates precisely what I have just described. Because porn is so powerful and lulls viewers so easily into a state of flow, it can commandeer resources that once kept other neurological pathways strong. Because of this, those pathways start to starve, degrade, and can eventually vanish.

Perhaps Joe Normal's business acumen starts to slip, or Joe Junior's baseball skills are slowly weathered away. The more time they spend watching porn, the stronger those sex superhighways become, adding new lanes and off-ramps while also putting up road-blocks, detours, or just tearing down old familiar but now seldom traveled roads.

Keep in mind that DeltaFosB is also responsible for creating triggers. Joe Normal and Joe Junior once had triggers to do all sorts of positive activities, but there is only so much room in their brains' hard drives. Since father and son are now watching porn instead of doing what they used to enjoy, their brains are overwriting the old triggers and adding replacements.

DeltaFosB is turning everything and anything into a trigger and rewiring their brains to crave porn.

This is the wired lock, in that these refashioned and newly-strengthened neurological pathways make sure the door remains wired shut.

There is more bad news. As Joe Normal and Joe Junior chase the dopamine high, CREB (meant to pump the brakes on the rush) is steadily building up in their brains. Over time, it's becoming harder and harder for them to feel that super heightened arousal that came so easily in the beginning.

Joe Normal and Joe Junior aren't watching porn for longer and longer periods of time just because they are slipping into flow. They are actually becoming numb to the experience, and it is taking longer and longer for them to become aroused and experience an orgasm. If father and son aren't already starting to see the early signs of erectile dysfunction, it is very likely on its way if they don't stop this addictive behavior.

The good news in all of this is that connections wired can also be rewired. It takes time, and because there are all the struggles that go with overcoming any addiction such as withdrawal, depression, mood swings, and cravings, it won't be easy. But thankfully, neuroplasticity is a two-way street. With work and dedication, we can replace bad roads with healthy ones simply by being mindful where we are allocating our mental and emotional resources.

The Habit Lock

For both Joe Normal and Joe Junior, there is a shift in behavioral patterns as their porn addictions intensify. DeltaFosB has turned a lot of everyday events, smells, senses, and feelings into cues to watch porn. The cue is coupled with a powerful craving and, like any powerful craving, Joe Normal and Joe Junior will deliberately start to make time for it. Life, activities, and interactions start being planned around online porn, because while the porn high is the addiction, checking out porn is becoming a habit. When I say a habit, I mean it is now a ritualized behavior they do automatically, like many of us might mindlessly check our Facebook or Instagram feeds.

Joe Normal once had his business, wife, and kids as the center of his world, and all other hobbies or activities orbited his core priorities. For Joe Junior, baseball, friends, school, a new girlfriend, and gaming once formed the center of his world, again with everything else orbiting around what he felt was most important. The epicenter of their worlds, however, are starting to shift fundamentally. Online porn is subtly becoming the sun around which everything else revolves.

All roads in their brains are starting to lead to porn. They might no longer even be consciously aware of what they are doing. Checking in on their favorite porn sites is as habitual as checking for text messages, emails, of even scrolling a social site. They get on their phones, computers, tablets, and the next thing they know, they are watching porn because this pattern has become so ingrained, it is no longer as noticeable because it's now as natural as riding a bike.

15

THE CAGE

T he entire internet has been chummed with bait. With its many challenges, struggles, and hardships, life can create triggers that tempt viewers to take the bait and step through the door. They are probably unaware of the locks that have been steadily squeezing their old lives out so they spend as much time and attention as possible in the Trap.

The Trap profits from their time, attention, and by devouring the viewers' lives. When we take the components of addiction, neurological rewiring, and habit forming, it is easy to see how viewers end up in the cage without realizing they are trapped. Even if the viewer has some sense that porn is becoming an addiction, it doesn't matter when so many perceived exits are actually overpasses designed to dump the viewer onto new roads that lead to different cages.

The Isolation Cage

We have talked about how the neurological pathways that get used the most are the ones that grow stronger. The problem with porn is that this is the pathway that grows increasingly stronger with every viewing, especially when it's paired with masturbation for orgasm.

Intimacy, arousal, connection, or even feeling loved used to be connected to pathways like talking, cuddling, hugging, or shared enjoyable activities that didn't necessarily have anything to do with sex.

Those healthy pathways that once ignited and strengthened all relationships, including friendships, are being dismantled. What is particularly problematic is that numerous neural pathways that once led to arousal—even something as simple as seeing the other partner or thinking of him or her—are steadily being demolished.

This same phenomenon is also happening to the adult entertainer, though in its mirrored opposite. All the pathways that once led to feelings of arousal, pleasure, and intimacy are being reconfigured as well. Sexual acts, even intimate acts like kissing, eventually become wired to negative feelings of exploitation, abuse, guilt, shame, and even pain. This is why many entertainers disassociate. Sex is no longer an act of love because it has been recoded as a form of assault. Assault is something to escape by disconnecting. This remapping of the brain is a main reason so many entertainers struggle with anxiety, depression, and substance abuse to help disconnect. This is also why so many are unable to forge healthy, loving relationships and gravitate to abusive ones, devoid of authentic intimacy. This remapped brain might possibly explain, at least in part, why so many who end up in adult entertainment were originally victims of sexual abuse and rape even before entering into the profession.

Back to the audience.

Porn paired with masturbation, over time, remaps the brain. Eventually, the viewer becomes physically unable to respond to old forms of stimulation such as kissing and other foreplay. Porn is now the only way he can become aroused and reach climax.

In the cases of Joe Normal and Joe Junior, I mentioned how the porn habit was already making them rearrange their lives and how they spent their time. They sought literal isolation to indulge in porn, but there are other levels in the isolation cage.

Thus far, my examples have been extreme because the Normal

family is trapped in a world that is anything but normal. With so many people's lives turned upside-down, porn has been big business during the pandemic, the best business probably ever. This said, though, there are other activities people can do even when they are mostly stuck at home. Joe Normal once spent time with his kids and his wife. They watched movies together or did little projects around the house. He chatted with friends online and talked to old business pals on LinkedIn. He would even shoot the breeze with his sons while he worked on that classic car in the garage, teaching them what he was doing and letting them help.

Joe Junior used to be active on social media. Even stuck inside, he interacted with schoolmates and friends via text. He might have played online video games, laughing and joking as he took on zombies with his buddies. Then, there was time with Dad and his brothers working on the car.

But porn is making both Joe Normal and Joe Junior pull away from everyone and everything. They are becoming steadily agitated, depressed, anxious, and alone, and not only because they are physically isolating. The pleasure they once felt hanging out with other people, with friends, or even in Joe Normal's case cuddling with his wife while they watched their favorite Netflix series in bed has faded. The neurological pathways that connected so many other people, places, events, and activities have been "saved over" by porn. What this means is that even in the presence of others, both father and son still feel detached and alone.

Let's set aside my extreme example of porn in a pandemic for now, because this process that leads to isolation was happening long before COVID-19. The pandemic might have simply made it worse because of forced confinement, limited activity, and unprecedented isolation. That, and any odd or negative mood changes could be easily blamed on other stressors. Others close to Joe Normal or Joe Junior might not realize there is a serious problem because so much else could be the cause of shortened tempers or self-isolation.

Let us say tomorrow everything reopens, and the world settles into a new normal. Joe Normal's wife returns to her high-paying job, and he is able to reopen his business. Maybe his business is doing better than ever because other people are going back to work, and other businesses are opening. People are tired of being cooped up and eager to be customers. Joe can also go back to the gym, meet his pals at the sports grill to watch a game, and return to church.

Joe Junior finally returns to school. He can hang out in person with his friends. He gets to play baseball again, and maybe his buddies tell him an even cuter girl than his first (and now ex) girlfriend has a crush on him.

Even if everything starts turning around for the better in a big way, Joe Normal and Joe Junior might not return to the people, hobbies, events, and activities they once loved because they have a new "love."

Porn.

The Fantasy Cage

Not only does porn lead to isolation, but it can also start to change tastes, preferences, and attitudes. Remember Nikolaas Tinbergen and his artificially enhanced butterflies? Tinbergen's cardboard creations demonstrate how butterfly behavior and human behavior are more alike than one might imagine. We already live in a culture that is saturated with supernormal stimuli, and it's having a noted impact on how people behave, especially when it comes to instinctual drives such as sex and reproduction.

Just flip through old magazines or watch some old movies. Many of the actors and actresses who were considered the gold standard of attractiveness back in the day would be lucky to be cast as an extra today. They certainly wouldn't be movie mega stars.

The standards for beauty have become so extreme that plastic surgery is so common as to be ordinary and even somewhat expected. Female models, actresses, and performers are all examples of the extreme. They are taller, thinner, with longer, thicker hair, pillow lips, round bottoms, large breasts, no extra fat, and never showing signs of age.

Compare a fifty-year-old female singer from the 1970s with J.Lo.

Males are not immune to these same pressures. Actors and models can range from thin to the point of being unhealthy to resembling a super beefed-up action figure more than a real human male. Adolescents and young men are struggling with every variety of body dysmorphia, a syndrome that has historically plagued females. These men may be starving themselves, or they are working out non-stop, taking steroids, and some are even getting implants in areas where they believe they are unable to grow enough muscle: pectorals, abs, glutes, quads, and so on. Their sense of what is normal has been skewed so far out of whack that it is almost impossible to live up to pop culture's standards of what it is to be desirable, or above normal.

And this is just the effect of regular everyday life, the ads, shows, magazines, and movies we all see, not porn.

In porn, everything—and I mean everything—is crazy-psychotic-mega-supernormal. Not only are male and female bodies are portrayed in their most extreme versions, but the sexual acts push every limit of the imagination. Porn storylines are meant to be completely and utterly over the top, even the so-called tame porn. Trust me, porn, by definition, is sex in a super-normal package. As we discussed in the first half of the book, real people don't have sex like this. **Men and especially women do not orgasm the way it is depicted in porn.** Keep in mind that the Trap is designed to thrive off head games and blurring the lines between reality and fantasy.

Women's bodies are not designed for the kind of physical trauma (which is the best word I can think of for it) that is portrayed even in the softest forms of porn. Male bodies aren't either. Most men do not have these massive penises. That, and a man who has sex for an hour or more without having an orgasm very likely has a physical problem. What is portrayed as normal in porn isn't anything real, healthy males should want to emulate. Gigantic penises are painful, even for porn actresses and actors. Sex that goes on for an hour or more is about as much fun for the sexual partner as being embraced by a jackhammer. Like the porn viewer, many male actors are so desensitized, they actually have difficulty reaching orgasm both on and off set.

Men of all ages are suffering terribly from immersing themselves in this fiction of a porn utopia. Their self-esteem plummets as fantasy overrides reality. Penile dysmorphic disorder (PDD) is not yet recognized by the Diagnostic and Statistical Manual as its own disorder, rather it is viewed as a subcategory of body dysmorphic disorder. This doesn't mean those experiencing PDD don't suffer terribly.[1] Their extreme anxiety about penis size or appearance causes severe anxiety, depression, and even suicidal thoughts. They might seek out risky, even shady, treatments and surgeries that can cause irreversible damage or even have life-threatening or life-ending outcomes.

According to the numbers, the rates of PDD seem to be increasing.[2] We can deduce this when we see the demand for penoplasty (penis enlargement surgery) is higher than ever and still climbing steadily. Is this a fluke and has nothing to do with porn? Perhaps. But I don't think so. According to the September 22, 2018, article by Colin Drury in the *Guardian*, "I Wanted a Truncheon in my Pants: the Rise of the Penis Extension,":

> *...between 2013 and 2017, members of the International Society of Aesthetic Plastic Surgery carried out 45,604 penis enhancements worldwide. Previous numbers are unknown; the procedure was considered such a minority concern that it wasn't included in surveys.[3]*

Think about that for a moment. There were so few penis enlargement surgeries performed before 2013, it was considered statistically insignificant. Then suddenly, this number skyrockets to almost 46,000 just in four years. Does it seem more than coincidental that this sudden demand for penis enlargement surgeries corresponds with when smartphones became affordable for the masses and online porn experienced its first waves of explosive growth?

I can tell you as a performer that this is no coincidence. Porn is destroying how men feel about their bodies, especially the size of their penises. Though I wanted to provide you with outsider references and expert testimony, the steady stream of emails I receive are nothing short of heartbreaking. I am constantly fielding messages about this very topic.

There are so many emails from men who are certain they are woefully small and inadequate that no woman would want them. I write countless messages assuring those who reach out that they are perfectly normal and actually desirable, telling them everything that I have packed into this book. I try to help them understand that porn is a lie, an illusion, and not to fall for it.

Men, young men and adolescents in particular, are already prone to anxiety about sex. Once they start using porn as the standard, however, they can begin to retreat more into fantasy because porn sets a bar they can never reach.

Porn distorts how they view their own desirability. They are terrified that a real flesh-and-blood partner wouldn't want them, so they willingly lock themselves away in the fantasy cage because of their irrational fear of rejection or even ridicule.

Normal, healthy ideas of sex are replaced with extremes. Viewers locked in the fantasy cage not only begin judging themselves more harshly, but others as well. Women in life don't look like the women in porn, neither do men. The viewers return to the source of supernormal stimulation, which is so much more exciting. If this goes on long enough, the viewer can no longer become physically aroused by anything but the supernormal: supernormal bodies and supernormal sexual acts.

In the world of online porn, there is limitless variety, and nothing in real life can compete. Since arousal and orgasm has been disconnected from actual intimacy, or a connection experienced with another person, eventually the viewer might begin dehumanizing those around him, particularly women.[4]

Females become sluts and whores, good for only one thing. The fantasy cage is the ideal environment for toxic masculinity to germinate and grow, unchecked and eventually out of anyone's control.

The Narcissist Cage

The narcissist cage shares a lot in common with the fantasy cage. Porn doesn't reflect real life, sex, or relationships, but as viewers consume more porn, they lose touch with truth and become more fixated on their own needs, wants, and desires.

The porn fantasy makes it seem that finding and pleasing a willing partner is effortless. That, and she will be always breathlessly awaiting her sex partner's attention and have no other priorities beyond her wanton desire to please. She will never be busy, tired, stressed, or have any needs that don't involve dropping everything to satisfy her sex partner's needs. All she will ever want is to provide increasingly wild adventures, complete with writhing, screaming orgasms. She never says no and is game for anything and everything.

If she has a bad day, isn't in the mood, can't orgasm just from penetration, or maybe requires something else like being held or having a conversation, clearly something is wrong with her. She is cold or needy. Perhaps, she doesn't want him at all and is rejecting him, maybe even cheating on him. Is she really not feeling well, or does she have her eye on someone else? He doesn't need this. She should be hungry to please, especially since she's no prize. The women in the videos are young, fit, and aren't letting themselves go.

The viewer who has stumbled into the narcissist cage develops a grossly distorted sense of how the partner should respond during sex, what she should want, and what she should be willing to do to satisfy her partner. Sex has become one-sided, and if the partner doesn't meet expectations, then the general idea is that she can be easily replaced.

According to the article, "Sexual Addiction: Insights from Psycho-analysis and Functional Neuroimaging," by Vincent Estellon & Harold Mouras:

> *Progressively, sexual excitement is increasingly distanced from the loving feelings associated with a relationship. The fact of loving implies both an encounter and sharing, loving someone else has the particular power of*

being able to tear a person away from a regressive position of narcissistic omnipotence in which he believes himself to be self-sufficient, capable of everything, all alone. If 'I can do everything all on my own,' I don't need anyone else.[5]

This is one of the many reasons that porn damages relationships, kills love, and cripples intimacy. The living, breathing partner becomes optional since the viewer is more aroused by what is online and can better satisfy himself.

What is truly saddening in this is that men do need love, intimacy, and connection as much as women. Porn warps this on both sides of the relationship. The partner can become worn out trying to please and meet expectations. Maybe she gives into the partner's demands, but he senses she is mentally checked out and is only going through the motions like a robot. Eventually the pair grows apart.

The Shame Cage

Sex is such a tricky subject all on its own. It's not a stretch to say that very few parents look forward to explaining to their children precisely how babies are made. American culture struggles with sex and we seem to find it difficult to separate sex and shame. This could be due to religion.

America has puritanical roots and, compared to Europe, is much more uncomfortable with nudity and sex. I was brought up Catholic, and trust me, we definitely never discussed sex other than it was sinful, an act shrouded in mystery, reserved for marriage and had something to do with making babies.

The problem, however, is empty space is still a place. If parents, guardians, educators, and institutions of faith remain silent about sex, then pop culture, peers, and porn will fill in the gaps. It is natural and healthy for children and young people to be curious about sex. Yet, when those who could be the most positive source for information are themselves ashamed of the subject, the problem only gets worse. Silence is a void that will get filled one way or another.

In chapter 12, we talked about how Joe Normal's watching of porn differed from Joe Junior's first time watching. Joe Junior's brain not only produced all the feel-good chemicals, but because this was foreign territory and his body was reacting in new and frightening ways, his brain also released cortisol. Our brains release cortisol when we are stressed and afraid.[6]

But the odds are actually quite high that Joe Normal's first encounter with sex was also from some kind of porn. Either he discovered his own dad's stash of magazines, or his buddies whisked him off someplace private to initiate him into the club. Maybe it was an adult, a family member, or neighbor.

Regardless, the chances are better than good that even Joe Normal associates sex with shame because of how he was first exposed. Because Dad associates sex with shame, he is unlikely to be the one to educate his son in a healthy manner. Thus, Joe Junior is initiated the same way, with the same formula that sex includes shame by default.

When sex and shame are packaged together this way, viewers are far more likely to view porn in secret. If, at some point, they realize they might possibly be addicted to it, they are stuck in a cage of shame and silence. Where can they turn to find someone who will listen?

The more the obsession takes hold, the stronger the shame cage becomes. Porn sites and porn advocates can claim all they want that sex is becoming less taboo and that people are more comfortable with sex than ever, but this doesn't necessarily translate into porn being a socially acceptable hobby, especially when it reaches a level of addiction.

Many of those addicted to porn are highly unlikely to admit they are struggling. While porn is something joked about, written off, and made light of, many porn-addicted people still feel a deep and profound shame. They might not only be ashamed for watching so much porn, but also disgusted by their own weakness and lack of willpower. They are mortified to admit they even need help to begin with, which makes sense. When celebrities like David Duchovny or

Tiger Woods release statements that they are checking into rehab to treat a "sex addiction," it suddenly becomes fodder for late night talk show jokes and internet memes. Maybe these celebrities are being disingenuous, but if they really are suffering from what we now see truly is a real and devastating problem, are we as a culture not compounding the issue and hampering their recovery with our ridicule and dismissiveness?

Since porn, like other addictions, requires increasingly stronger doses over time to reach the same high, many trapped in this cycle are no longer stimulated by normal porn and have already started the decline into kinkier, weirder, more extreme and violent porn. This only makes the situation worse, reinforcing the bars on the shame cage.

It might be one thing for Joe Normal to admit to a counselor that he is addicted to porn, but it is another order of magnitude entirely for him to be fully transparent with his wife and family in a way that could lead to actual help and healing. How can he muster the courage to admit that he can only be aroused watching women humiliated, raped, or brutalized? How does he confess that he is numb unless the videos feature entertainers who at least appear to be underage or look like children? What if he has become consumed watching videos featuring the most fringe fetishes like extreme torture, bestiality, or snuff films?

This would require him to admit he has something worse than a porn addiction. From his perspective, he would have to admit he is a sadist, a misogynist, a budding pedophile, a deviant freak, or what-ever shameful label he now has attached to his identity. How could he not dread the pain his admission could cause? His wife might very well see his behavior as tantamount to cheating. He is afraid he might lose authority over his kids and that they will never respect or trust anything he has to say, let alone anything about sex.

Self-loathing, guilt, and isolation only add more fuel to the inferno that is burning away any bridges that might lead to escape, healing, and restoration.

Kindness is the Key to Unlock the Cages

With each of these chapters, I want to offer a sense of hope and that there are answers to these vastly complex problems. We can change this, take control, and make it better if we are willing to do the hard work.

The Trap and all its cages have a critical weakness: kindness. Throughout this entire book, I have mentioned over and over how shame plays a key role on both sides of the issue, for performers and addicts alike.

For those who have been unfortunate enough to find themselves trapped in a porn addiction and are aware they have hurt others they care about, shame is a major barrier. This is a hurdle for every addiction, though. But I want to point out that there is a fundamental difference between shame and guilt.

Dr. Brené Brown, author of the *New York Times* best-selling book *Daring Greatly,* said it brilliantly in her blog post January 14, 2013, blog post "Shame v. Guilt,":

> *Based on my research and the research of other shame researchers, I believe that there is a profound difference between shame and guilt. I believe that guilt is adaptive and helpful—it's holding something we've done or failed to do up against our values and feeling psychological discomfort.*
>
> *I define shame as the intensely painful feeling or experience of believing that we are flawed and therefore unworthy of love and belonging—something we've experienced, done, or failed to do makes us unworthy of connection.*[7]

Based on this interpretation, we see that guilt is a sense that a behavior is wrong and needs to be replaced with something better, healthier. Shame, on the other hand, attaches a label to a person, with the person and the behavior becoming one and the same.

As an example, say a person cheated on their spouse. They feel guilty. After a time, they can't live this way any longer, want to come clean, and make things right. Admitting they were unfaithful, being able to go through the process of confession, and asking for forgiveness are already extremely hard. They are exposed and at the mercy of the person(s) they wronged, hoping that will be willing to forgive them and possibly give them another chance. Retaliation, rejection, the thought of being banished from family or social groups, or even fears of eternal damnation all cement shame in place. Kindness can ease the addict's genuine concerns about coming clean.

The guilty person accepts responsibility for their failings. This person longs to do the necessary steps to rebuild trust, and, in time, undo the damage. In this instance, restoration is possible because guilt is a motivation for change. Guilt is what says, "My behavior was wrong, and I know I can do better. No, I *will* do better." Shame is drastically different. Guilt is: "I cheated." Shame is: "I am a cheater." Guilt offers a path to redemption, whereas shame declares the person is the behavior and therefore will never be worthy of forgiveness, love, or connection.

Kindness short-circuits shame. It permits all parties to express their hurt and process guilt and forgiveness without marking the person who has fallen with indelible ink reading, "Damaged Goods."

Porn is a very complex subject. For many who watch porn, they might never find themselves at this point. Yet, there are many who do. When it comes to porn addiction, shame is totally counterproductive, as is the case when dealing with any addiction. Guilt, however, allows a person to examine what they have become wrapped up in. Does the dehumanization, objectification, or even violence toward others for sexual pleasure align with their values or the values they want to have? Does this fit with their long-term relationship goals? If not, then guilt can propel them to seek help, and kindness from others can help them undo the locks and help set the addict on the path to healing and freedom.

16

THE CHAINS THAT BIND

When talking about online porn, the viewer can expect many different varieties of chains that bind them to their compulsion. There are physical, psychological, emotional, and digital chains. In ways, the chains that bind porn viewers are more complex than those that ensnare the adult entertainer, and we will go through these one by one.

Physical Chains

To an extent, we have already addressed some of these physical chains. Though obviously not every person who watches porn is doomed to tumble off the cliff of addiction, many do. The porn addict starts watching more porn to chase the initial high. It takes longer to feel arousal because CREB has built up in the brain.

They can't seem to focus on anything else because DeltaFosB has refashioned their world into a web of cues signaling that it is time to go watch porn. Like any addiction, the decreasingly satisfying highs are followed by deeper and darker lows, so the viewer keeps returning to porn to self-medicate and self-soothe.

The images they see might cause a plummet in self-esteem, lead to penile dysmorphic disorder (PDD), and cause the viewer to steadily isolate which only makes the situation worse. But there is another consequence that can also be devastating to males. The sharp rise of online porn viewership seemingly correlates with a sharp rise in erectile dysfunction and low libido in males.[1]

Shockingly, this disorder is now having a serious impact on males under the age of twenty-five, who, until the past several years, have historically represented almost a statistically insignificant group. This sharp rise in cases of erectile dysfunction appeared right around the time online porn became readily accessible, making it tough to dismiss as at least one correlative, if not causal factor.

Erectile dysfunction, until recent decades, was usually a disorder that impacted older males due to physical reasons directly related to aging: low testosterone, obesity, diabetes, heart conditions, etc. Though these are still factors for erectile dysfunction, some researchers are now inclined to believe the limitless novelty and unfettered accessibility of online porn combined with its impact on the brain might play a significant role as well.

Some experts believe men are no longer dealing with simple erectile dysfunction. Mounting evidence is leading some researchers at least to consider porn among major contributing factors. As a result, the concept of porn-induced erectile dysfunction, or PIED,[2] is attracting more medical and scientific scrutiny. Researchers are finding that, while many men can attain an erection while watching porn, they cannot attain or maintain one with a physical partner. This then leads to more distancing from an actual mate or partner. Additionally, since the brain is designed to seek out the novel, and online porn has millions of hours of novelty to offer, men are gravitating more and more to self-gratification using porn. Without porn, their bodies won't cooperate because a normal partner cannot offer the super dopamine hit that the supernormal images porn can.

According to an academic article in the *MDPI Behavioral Sciences Journal,* "Is Internet Pornography Causing Sexual Dysfunctions? A Review with Clinical Reports,":

When a user has conditioned his sexual arousal to Internet pornography, sex with desired real partners may register as 'not meeting expectations' (negative reward prediction) resulting in a corresponding decline in dopamine. Combined with the inability to click to more stimulation, this unmet prediction may reinforce an impression that partnered sex is less salient than Internet pornography use.

Internet pornography also offers a voyeur's perspective generally not available throughout partnered sex. It is possible that if a susceptible Internet pornography user reinforces the association between arousal and watching other people have sex on screens while he is highly aroused, his association between arousal and real-life partnered sexual encounters may weaken.[3]

If we go back to Joe Normal and Joe Junior, both father and son are potentially at risk for suffering erectile dysfunction. Joe Normal already has enough stress on his plate and is struggling with his sense of being a man since he believes he has failed his wife and family as a provider. Now, one of the most fundamental measurements of his masculinity or virility is also failing him when he tries to have sex with his wife. Their marriage suffers even more because they no longer have sex. He can't perform, and thus Joe Normal's shame spiral only gains more momentum.

As for the son, Joe Junior is young and already bombarded with confusion around sex. He might once have gotten an erection simply by seeing his old girlfriend's picture, or even while chatting online with a cute girl from school. He once felt the tingles and chills that skittered all over his body. But now, there is nothing. He feels empty. When suddenly he realizes he can't feel those tingles and chills, or get an erection outside of porn, this only adds more fear to the cocktail that was brimming with enough fear to begin with. It also adds in a healthy dose of shame and more self-loathing. He is a teenager. He is supposed to be a horndog twenty-four seven! What is wrong with him? Will he need to get a pill to get hard like some old man?

Porn addiction does affect the body, because how can it not? If porn rewires the brain, and the brain guides libido as well as the sex organs, then it only seems logical if there is a genuine link between porn addiction and erectile dysfunction. If a person chasing a constant high from increasingly tantalizing or shocking porn scenarios is *simultaneously* becoming numb to anything reality has to offer, this is a serious concern.

I know this is a controversial claim, but I can attest that this is a real problem. I have worked as an adult entertainer for enough years to see this phenomenon firsthand. Men who became increasingly hooked on porn eventually needed more extreme scenarios to attain and maintain an erection and achieve orgasm. Over time, even that didn't work. Many had to rely on medications to be able to get an erection. They started seeking out personal webcamming sessions with me, since watching my films was no longer enough. Then, as time went on, the webcamming scenarios changed as well. They began requesting more bizarre and increasingly violent storylines. I could tell these men were moody, dark, and depressed. Some even confessed how they couldn't enjoy actual sex with another partner anymore, compounding the stress and hopelessness they felt.

Yes, my claims are anecdotal, but I have been on the front lines. No, I am not a doctor, but I do have a nursing degree, so I know sound science when I read it. However, beyond the research papers and clinical trials, I can't deny what I have witnessed for years happen time and time again. Remember the client who wanted me to cover myself in bullet holes and pretend to be dying while he got off? He didn't start out that way. Once that story wouldn't work, where could he go from there? What is the next level of extreme that could arouse him?

But let's back up a bit. How do viewers find themselves trapped in such darkness in the first place?

Shadow Chains

For many years I could not, for the life of me, understand this progression. Why were audiences seeming to go off the metaphorical deep end of porn? What was driving them from regular porn to craving storylines that were so violent, cruel, or depraved? Why would they even find that appealing?

I have personally observed this sort of change during my twenty-year tenure as an entertainer. Over time, many viewers realize they can only get aroused watching material that previously they would have deemed disgusting, cruel, immoral, unethical, or even criminal. Other studies have recorded another darker and perhaps more insidious shift. These viewers aren't merely aroused by scenarios that once would have repulsed them, but they start believing these behaviors are more common than they really are and are even completely acceptable.

There is one famous experiment that expertly demonstrates how this shift can happen.

Like most of us humans, rats, too, are naturally repelled by the smell of death. A researcher named Jim Faust was curious if this natural instinct to avoid death could be overridden and devised an experiment to prove his theory.[4] He placed virgin male rats in a cage with female rats who had been sprayed with a substance that emulated the stench of a dead, rotting rat.

This was when things started to get odd.

For the males, their desire to mate overpowered their aversion to the smell and they coupled with partners that should have sent them scurrying. This was bizarre for sure, but not nearly as strange as what Faust later discovered. He placed the male rats in cages with dowel rods to play with, some soaked in the same chemical that smelled like a dead, rotting rat. To his shock, he observed that the male rats actually preferred to play with the objects that smelled of death. Why?

Good question.

As we have already discussed, during sex the brain releases a massive rush of dopamine. Thus, Faust reasoned that when the rats had sex, they associated the pleasurable experience of sex with the smell of death. Changing the rats' experience and attaching it to a new and formerly detestable association was powerful enough to completely override their natural instinct.

The article, "Instant Transformation of Learned Repulsion into Motivational 'Wanting,'" goes into deeper detail on this phenomenon.[5]

One might be tempted to protest at this point. *Hey, we are humans, not dumb rats!* True. We drive cars, have smartphones, and some of us even own fondue pots. Yet, when we get down to the basics, humans, like rats, are mammals, and all mammals have fairly similar reward centers. And these reward centers are vulnerable to being warped.

The rats had their Faustian sex bargain, just as we humans have our own.

Since we have dedicated a lot of time to discussing addiction, you already know that someone who is becoming more reliant on porn naturally is prone to gravitate to increasingly extreme, shocking, or outrageous content either from curiosity or because they eventually become numb to the tamer content. They need more for the same fix, to experience that super heightened arousal. But they don't always end up in the shadowy corners of porn all on their own. Sometimes, they have help.

Hidden Hands that Tug the Chains

Always keep in mind that software operating behind the scenes is programmed to keep viewers online, watching and engaging as long as possible. Many online porn sites not only pillaged the casino play-book, but they also pillaged the same tools that most of the social media sites rely on to improve engagement.

This means one of the programs' prime directives is to curate content intelligently. Content curation maximizes the odds the viewer will not only keep returning, but also slip into the machine zone quicker, thus remaining longer and longer on the site. Remember those self-evolving smart algorithms? The software can tell when Joe Normal or Joe Junior stop paying as much attention. Maybe they didn't finish watching a video, or they left the site to do something else. When it comes to business and making money, that is a problem, but it's one the software can fix by using all that raw data and the viewers' algorithmic identities.

By cross-indexing Joe Normal's and Joe Junior's algorithmic identities with similar users, the site's software can better predict what kind of content it needs to slip into their feeds to prod them back to paying attention again. What worked on other viewers algorithmically similar to Joe Normal? What worked on other viewers similar to Joe Junior?

Back in chapter 10, I mentioned the paper, "Desire by Design: Pornography as Technology Industry," by Patrick Keilty. I will parse out the section most useful for what we are discussing now:

> *These designers are responsible for making strategic choices about information management and the graphical organization of content that translates into large profits, innovative capitalist media techniques, and dominant modes for curating, distributing, and regulating our experience of sexual desire today.*[6]

Notice how Keilty mentions graphical organization. This is extremely important. When we are online, there is a sense that we are choosing what we are watching.

As the joke goes, we hop on YouTube to check out one video and five hours later find ourselves watching a detailed tutorial on how to communicate with giraffes. The content that flows into our feed isn't haphazard or accidental. It is selected deliberately not to serve you, the viewer, but to bring you as a viewer in-line with serving a corporate goal.

Online porn sites are outfitted with some of the world's most advanced data-mining software. Unless Joe Normal or Joe Junior take certain precautions to hide their data and online activity, it's a fairly reasonable conclusion that this software can mine what Joe Normal and Joe Junior search for, watch, look at, and respond to even when they aren't watching porn. Using that mined data, the software can then modify accordingly to queue up content that might not only hook them into watching, but also keep them watching.

The longer viewers remain engaged on the site, the more valuable they become. More time on the site not only offers more time for critical data-mining, but the longer audiences watch, the more ads they will see. And, as should be fairly clear by now, consumer profiles developed using "random" raw data and ad revenues are where the real money is made.

The Invisible Chains

Some of you reading might think this is all a bit far-fetched, but we take a lot of the online experience for granted. We don't know how it works, and many of us don't bother asking because it's either intimidating or boring or both. We don't care how our favorite sites work so long as they give us what we want...or even what we never knew we wanted.

Perhaps you hopped online and searched for information about diabetes because your mom was just diagnosed. Then, lo and behold, guess what appears almost immediately in the sidebar on Facebook: ads for insulin and diabetic supplies and supplements. How did they know? You were on a totally different website!

This is surveillance capitalism at work, and it is so pervasive that it has become invisible, like a subroutine. We don't even notice it, not really, because it's everywhere and always there. When we do notice the telltale signs of surveillance capitalism, we might even think it isn't that big of a deal. In fact, it makes life easier because, unlike the old days, we are no longer flooded with ads that aren't relevant. The "spray and pray" days when advertisers blasted out mass messages and hoped some hit the right target are gone.

There are many reasons why this covert data mining should bother us, but I am only going to focus on how this practice is relevant to online porn. The people and companies behind online porn sites understand the psychology of keeping users hooked. But these sites need massive amounts of information to make the psychological levers work effectively. Enter: data-mining.

We can use Joe Normal as an example of how hidden hands can use the invisible chains to nudge his online behavior. Once Joe clicks on the free porn, if he keeps watching over longer periods of time, we know that it's highly probable his tolerance for the milder porn eventually will build up. He might then start seeking harder forms of porn on his own. This is why porn sites rely on possessing those massive reservoirs of every kind of content imaginable. They want to make sure that there is more than enough material to keep Joe logged in and turned on as much as possible.

But there is a second scenario. Joe Normal's interest in what he is currently watching flags because, "Sorority Girls Gone Wild," simply doesn't do it for him anymore. But Joe has lived a rather strait-laced life and wouldn't know what else to search for. That, or maybe his strict religious upbringing keeps him from actively seeking out more hardcore content on his own. This is when a site's algorithms step in to give him a nudge and tug those invisible chains a bit, guiding him where they need him to go to keep him watching. The site then applies Joe's algorithmic identity to slip in content Joe might have never looked for if left to fend for himself.

The site already knows he watches porn, duh. But what else does the software know? His data profile indicates that he is middle aged, white, heterosexual, having marriage trouble (someone searched for online couple's therapy on his computer). Earlier in the week, he refilled a prescription for a strong antidepressant as well as a new anti-anxiety med through his pharmacy's website. Joe used to watch race car shows, but in the past month, he has replaced those shows with pre-COVID-19 MMA fight videos. His resumé is on at least ten different sites, but the analytics show he has not gotten much if any response.

The software also indicates he has recently been streaming a lot of extremist political shows and was put in Facebook jail for trolling. Joe's credit score has plunged in a few short months, his credit cards are all maxed out, and data indicates he listed his classic car for sale on a local website over the weekend. With just these snippets of information, it doesn't take a genius or even a particularly smart algorithm to see that Joe Normal is probably a toxic soup of pent-up aggression.

This online information was once considered digital trash back in the days when Google was just getting off the ground. Back then, it was worthless, mostly because it existed as scattered and disconnected bits of data. But now this digital detritus is collected, sorted, and molded into an eerily revealing profile that algorithms can then use to adjust the videos they have been slotting into Joe Normal's feed. The next time he logs on, the algorithms use all of this information to self-correct and modify his content curation. Why not slip in some mild S&M into his video feed to see if he will click? Bingo! According to the analytics, Joe Normal not only clicked, but he kept watching most of the night. Even better, Joe's visits have been steadily increasing in number as well as duration since the shift in content.

Any time Joe's attention wanes, the algorithms adjust and simply suggest something even more outrageous. Shock value alone is a good hook, but Joe Normal is one ticked-off dude. The algorithms continue to tweak and evolve to maximize the desired outcome, i.e., Joe's time. It might eventually insert titles like "Punish the Bitches," "Filthy Whores Get What's Cumming," then "Dirty Slut Smackdown," and it's jackpot! Joe's visits are lasting longer than ever. He has even started to click on the paid services in spite of the fact that he is broke.

Maybe now it's a bit clearer how we might not be so different from those deranged death rats after all. Six months earlier when Joe Normal couldn't sleep and clicked on free porn, it's safe to assume he didn't think it was any big deal. In fact, it should be less of a deal than when he sneaked in to check out his dad's stash of *Playboy* magazines because he is no longer a kid. He is a grown man. He didn't think there was any harm in it. In fact, he had the best sex he'd had in ages with his wife later that night, didn't he?

If anyone had asked him after that first encounter if he enjoyed watching women being beaten, raped, and sodomized by large groups of masked men, he probably would have been offended or even horrified.

Yet here he is.

What are the odds that Joe will be able to maintain a strict long-term separation between his beliefs and the online world? If he is filling his head with rape scenarios, torture, exploitation, and degradation, it's reasonable to conclude that watching hours and hours of violent misogyny could start coloring how he views females in general.

Remember the rats and how they felt the dopamine rush when coupled with sex as well as the smell of death? What about when Joe Normal feels the dopamine rush of an orgasm from hearing a woman cry out in pain, beg for mercy, or struggle to break free? He feels the rush when he sees a woman being yelled at, punched, kicked, called names, and sexually brutalized. Just like the male rats associated the smell of death with something positive, the same phenomenon can happen to Joe Normal. What once repelled him—a female being harmed—has the very real potential to be rewired by his own brain as something attractive and enticing. Like the male rats that gravitated to the dowel rods that reeked of death and ignored the normal playthings, Joe Normal is heading into extremely treacherous territory of escalating behaviors.

This said, humans are vastly complex. There is no simple formula because every viewer is completely unique. Not every person who watches hardcore violent porn is destined to become a misogynist, rapist, or sadosexual serial killer. Such a gross oversimplification is absurd. While we know that not every person who drinks a beer is doomed to become a hopeless alcoholic, we still insist on warning labels. When it comes to prescription medications, if even a statistically insignificant percentage of people have experienced a negative side-effect, by law, that negative side-effect must be listed.

When it comes to online porn, algorithms can and do nudge viewers down certain paths they might never have found on their own. This is the insidious nature of online porn in particular. I keep repeating that technology doesn't have a conscience, but the people who design are responsible for all aspects of software design do, or, maybe at least they should.

Online porn isn't the first industry that has put profit ahead of all consequences. Western civilization has always battled robber barons who placed money above human life, public safety, the environment, etc. We have taken on companies who strip-mined, clear-cut forests, polluted the air and water, knowingly sold toxic products to trusting consumers, and who had no concern for worker safety or public health. The push for revenue without responsibility is why, at least in the United States, we now have the Environmental Protection Agency (EPA), Occupational Safety and Hazard Administration(OSHA), Food and Drug Administration(FDA), Federal Trade Commission (FTC), and many others.

I get that much of the software and algorithms are machines and thus neutral. They are only sending viewers like Joe Normal to the places his data profile indicates he might want to go. He is an adult, so who are they to censor what he wants?

Maybe they have a point.

But what about Joe Junior? Do these sites get to hide behind free speech and protections afforded by Section 230 of the Communications Decency Act when it comes to minors? Can they argue that their software is morally neutral and therefore they have no responsibility? I mean, they did include a box to make viewers pinkie promise to be eighteen or older, right? This is a real issue because Joe Junior's data profile might also include a lot of the markers that ping the algorithms to curate his feed much the same way as his father's.

How do we feel about a teenage boy accessing a site that not only normalizes rape and violence, but links misogyny with sexual arousal? Are we okay with, as *Bitdefender* reported, the fact that the sites most visited by children under the age of 10 featured categories such as "extreme brutal gang bang," "sleep assault," "domestic discipline," and "crying in pain?"[7]

It's a question worth asking.

Addiction Chains

If the main goal is to hook viewers using free content in hopes they will eventually opt in for the paid services, this is a financial win for the site, but what about the user? I have already detailed how porn addiction, like any other addiction, can be an escalating behavior. These sites are counting on this because when audiences venture over to the paid services, there is a higher return on investment.

According to John Schwartz's article in the *New York Times*, "The Pornography Industry vs. Digital Pirates," Wendy Seltzer, an attorney and fellow at Yale University, said, "Seeing [free porn] just whets their appetite for more," Seltzer said. "Once they get through what's available for free, they'll move into the paid services."[8]

This is not an unusual business practice. Some internet television channels such as Hulu offer an option that's free but filled with ads. You have a choice, however, to upgrade to the paid ad-free version. Freemium gaming runs on the same model. My point is that offering something free in hopes that it will lead to paying for a service is nothing unusual.

In light of so much evidence that porn can be addictive, the dynamic between porn dealer and porn consumer might also resemble a drug dealer offering the first few hits free. The dealer is aware not everyone will become an addict. Any losses the dealer may take handing out free products are more than made up for by that certain percentage who become addicted and thus regular customers. What's even better is a portion of those customers will become hardcore addicts, the most loyal and high-paying clientele ever to exist.

Porn exists in this odd limbo between these two poles. Their business model hovers in the gray areas.

Digital Chains

The internet is still very much a digital Wild West. There is a lot of uncharted territory, unknown dangers, and it is easy to be lulled into a false sense of safety online. Digital chains can trip up porn viewers in a myriad of ways.

Ironically, many of the digital chains that snag so many adult performers into the Trap can also grab hold of viewers. Not only is everything on the internet forever, but we are not always in control of what content is posted.

Online activity always leaves a trail, a chain of activity that can be traced to a user. These chains can be exploited in any number of ways, but ultimately, they are powerful enough to seal even viewers into the box.

17

THE BOX

When discussing the Trap, the performers boxes might vary from that of the viewer, but it's still a box, and the end result for anyone in this deep is rarely good. For the audience, online porn sites have chummed the waters with a wide variety of bait. These companies know everyone has triggers but also that there is no such thing as one bait-hook-fits-all.

Once a site dangles the right bait that leads a viewer through the door, then any number of locks can materialize to secure the viewer inside the cage. For good measure, the chains that bind act as a redundancy measure for securing the audience inside this fantasy world until it becomes the box.

The box differs from the cage in that the person is completely sealed up. The cage had bars. One could peer into the outside world. The box, however, is a world of walls. Fantasy and reality fuse together and escape is much harder.

As we discussed in the first half of the book, many webcammers believed they were making extra money performing a private session for a client, only to later find that private session was posted on some online porn site. These entertainers didn't choose to become porn

stars. Someone else made the choice for them without their knowledge or consent. Ah, but what can happen on one side of the screen
can happen on the other. This means that the audience, just like the
adult entertainer, could end up trapped in a box not of their making.

The Porn Box

The client who trusted he was participating in a private session could
very well find that intimate experience uploaded for all the world to
see. As we have seen, once that content goes live, the damage can't be
undone even if the victim manages to get the video taken down on
one site.

If Joe Normal thought getting a job was tough before, imagine the
fallout if a shady webcamming company posts his session on a porn
site? Maybe the webcamming company is actually blameless and
kept his information private. What if the company was hacked and
the clients threatened with exposure or doxing?

It's not as if something similar hasn't happened before.
Remember the Ashley Madison scandal?

*In July 2015, a group calling itself 'The Impact Team' stole the user data of
Ashley Madison, a commercial website billed as enabling extramarital
affairs. The group copied personal information about the site's user base
and threatened to release users' names and personally identifying
information if Ashley Madison would not immediately shut down.*[1]

When Ashley Madison refused to comply, the group made good
on their threat and leaked more than sixty gigabytes of the company's
data, including user's personal information.[2]

Joe Normal might unwittingly end up a porn star, or find himself
publicly outed in Ashley Madison fashion. No site is impenetrable;
thus, anything is possible. The damage to his marriage, family, and
reputation could be ruinous. If he had hoped to reopen his business
or get a new job, he now has a much steeper and far more treach-

erous mountain to climb. He is left to endure very public humiliation and all that goes with the Scarlet XXX.

What's worse, his family is branded with the same scorn and shame as well. His wife might lose her friends, her small business, her security clearance, or her job. What if she teaches small children? It isn't beyond the bounds of possibility that the PTA will readily line up with pitchforks and torches and demand her resignation. She is a deviant by association! As for Joe Junior, he could become a pariah among his peers, as well as among adults. What parent wants their kid hanging out with...*that* kid? The apple doesn't fall far from the tree, you know.

Joe Normal may be shunned by family, neighbors, church members, potential investors, employers, clients, and customers. His son returns to school and resumes playing baseball. Even though Joe Normal has done nothing illegal, even though he was the victim, it won't matter. Odds are better than good that he will be boxed into the same category as a sex offender, or at least a pervert no one wants their kids or partner around...exactly like adult entertainers. Oh, the irony.

Exposure is only one of many pitfalls that viewers face when tangling with the Trap.

I already pointed out one cultural hypocrisy. There seems to be this unwritten rule that it's acceptable to watch porn, just not to do porn. There is another hypocrisy that impacts the audience. It is acceptable to watch porn so long as no one finds out about it.

If our society really is as progressive and accepting of adult entertainment as many pundits and porn sites would like us to believe, then why would viewers risk backlash if their private porn activity were suddenly made public information? Perhaps there are some reading this who truly believe such dire repercussions are unfair and unjust. What a consenting adult does in private shouldn't be weaponized against them, especially when they haven't done anything against the law.

This is true, but if we look at the fallout from the Ashley Madison data breach, it's plain to see that fair is only a weather condition. Cheating on one's partner isn't illegal, but many Ashley Madison "offenders" soon found themselves thrust into the court of public opinion where the public punishment meted out far outweighed the perceived private crime.

Charles Orlando's investigative article, "I Was Hacked on Ashley Madison — But It's You Who Should Be Ashamed," provides unsettling insight into the modern mob mentality:

> But perhaps the most disturbing trend is the condescending judgment of those who can't wait for the cheaters to face public humiliation and be outed. I'm not an advocate for infidelity, but it's shockingly sad to see so many people lying-in-wait for the certain destruction of many lives. Marriages might end and children are about to find out about their parents' exploits online. The hackers are offering vigilante justice, and the mob that is the Internet is more than willing to serve as judge, jury, and executioner.
>
> People are hungrily waiting to punish members of Ashley Madison with public humiliation, which is alarming.
>
> These aren't people who put the public in danger ... they're having a private affair (or at least trying to have one). How is this worthy of public shaming? It seems to me that these people definitely have some explaining to do to their significant other, but they don't deserve a flogging in the virtual town square with millions of onlookers.[3]

It's precisely because of this sort of public shaming that numerous suicides as well as cases of extortion and reports of hate crimes followed in the wake of the data breach.[4]

Many who engage in adult entertainment services, such as private webcamming sessions, haven't done anything illegal. Those legally old enough to watch porn haven't broken any laws either. One might say that it's their private life, so no big deal.

The problem is that nothing online is private. Nothing online is safe, not now or ever. As Charles Orlando points out in the same article from above:

No matter what any site guarantees, if you post it ... it's out there. You might as well be standing on a hilltop screaming whatever you just posted — or drank, or smoked, or did in a dungeon with three other people and a photographer wearing a panda suit.[5]

When discussing adult entertainment, it would be tough to argue that if this private activity were made public that nothing bad would happen. Many users on Ashley Madison exchanged intimate messages, described detailed fantasies, and swapped scandalous images. Some never physically cheated. Some weren't even members of the site, but that made little difference once everything was out for all to see and judge. The social media and internet bloodhounds weren't about to wait and verify if the leaked information had been vetted. They were too eager for the hunt. If the members of Ashley Madison experienced this sort of major blowback, then one can make the logical assumption that porn viewers could be taking similar life-altering risks.

Again, my role here isn't to take sides as much as it is to shine a light on some very hard, shadowy truths. The idea that there is nothing wrong with a consenting adult watching porn and imbibing in online porn services doesn't withstand the test of reality. It's too easy for a viewer to end up trapped in the porn box, facing the same public excoriation as adult entertainers and porn stars, maybe even far worse.

I have been trapped in the porn box for years and am all too familiar with the relentless onslaught of those who have an opinion about me and need me to know about it. If you have read this far, you also know how many times I tried to escape this line of work but failed. The Scarlet XXX was simply too prominent. But the public knows I have been a career adult entertainer for years. There is no gotcha.

For our imaginary Joe Normal, the gavel strike might come down harder should, say, a private webcamming session get uploaded for all to see. It could even be tougher for Joe Normal because, unlike a porn star, Joe dared present himself as an upstanding citizen, business owner, husband, father, but then others found out the truth. Sadly, the court of public opinion is one of the most brutal and unforgiving.

The Violated Box

I believe the previous section made it pretty clear that we are all vulnerable once we venture online. There is a reason it is a good idea to change our passwords regularly, whether that is on social media, online banking, or shopping on websites. Those who visit porn sites know, or at least really should know, that these places are brimming with malware, viruses, phishers, hackers, etc.

If Joe Normal did not properly secure his computer, which is almost impossible to do anyway, then he has left himself open to being hacked, doxed, extorted, or having his computer locked down by ransomware. Every time he gets online, he leaves digital fingerprints on all the pages he visits. Most of the internet relies on a system called, "http," (hypertext transfer protocol) for the transfer of information. Recently, a new system, https (s standing for "secure") has been widely adopted to protect information by encoding it. However, many porn sites, especially ones offering free porn, aren't upgraded to the new https, so anyone browsing a porn site is opening a gateway for hackers to gain access to all kinds of personal information like credit card numbers and passwords.

Viewing porn using a public Wi-Fi network is just begging for trouble because it doesn't even take a skilled hacker to obtain access to personal information. In spite of the dangers, there has been a sharp rise in audiences logging in to view porn at work, or using free access afforded by libraries, universities, coffee shops, airports, and more.

All this to say that Joe Normal's maxed out credit cards and plummeting credit score might not have even been due to his own poor money management. Joe very well could be the victim of identity theft. What is possibly more unsettling is that Joe Normal might not have even been the source of the problem. Maybe he did take certain precautions, but did his fifteen-year-old son know to do the same? Joe Junior may have been clever enough to use the elderly neighbor's Wi-Fi and savvy enough to erase his browser history. But was he also aware of the digital dangers that can come with clicking certain links or downloading content from particular sites? Did he understand the perils of public Wi-Fi?

By this point, some might argue that surfing porn using incognito or private mode offered by most browsers provides total privacy. But again, total privacy is a myth. In an interview on *Vice*, "Your Porn is Watching You," Justin Brookman, a privacy expert at the Center for Democracy & Technology, asserted that incognito mode does:

> ...[v]irtually zero to stop this tracking, and at best your address bar won't auto-complete to something embarrassing, but advertisers and data brokers still get the information. I have no idea what, if anything, they do with it—but it's all sitting in a database somewhere.[6]

Experts disagree about the consequences that go with surfing porn in incognito mode. Opinions vary from this being a formula to be hacked/extorted/your-life-is-ruined to no-big-deal and you might simply start seeing more ads for bustiers and leather outfits. Just know that most workplaces, government agencies and any company doing a decent background check can see where a viewer has been, even while incognito. This might mean the difference between a hiring or firing, gaining or losing security clearance, or getting a promotion versus a pink slip.

Thus, if we want to maintain the argument that porn has no impact on everyday life, maybe it doesn't. Maybe the risk of addiction isn't a significant risk. Experts do disagree as to whether or not, and to what extent or not, porn poses a threat to mental health, relationships, and altered behavior.

This said, I side with the research that reflects what I have personally witnessed over the past two decades. I have literally witnessed people change—and not for the better—once immersed in or addicted to porn. Not only did I deal with this early in life with my first husband, but I also couldn't even count how many fans I have seen slip into increasingly negative attitudes, behaviors, and thought patterns.

But, for those who believe online porn is harmless, that is your prerogative, and we can agree to disagree. However, it's fairly tough to deny that even a casual online porn viewer chances ending up in the violated box. Online porn sites pose significant security threats, and there is a very real danger a viewer could have his identity stolen, computers and devices corrupted, or personal information leaked.

Again, my role here is simply to offer awareness. Those of legally consenting age can weigh the risks versus threats. If, however, we refer back to that stat *Bitdefender* provided indicating that 1 out of every 10 online porn viewers under the age of 18 was 10 years old or younger, the big picture shifts dramatically.[7]

It's a fairly safe bet that a young child isn't overly concerned or even truly aware that he has just opened a potentially catastrophic and life-altering data breach by sneaking a peek at weird fetish porn on Nana's computer while she was babysitting him. The child wants to sneak another peek at what his friends showed him on the bus. He is curious. In this scenario, Nana wasn't even part of the porn audience, but she might very well suffer a lot of needless hardship. Because online porn has virtually no barriers to entry, her young grandson can unintentionally open her life to every sort of cyberattack.

The Reality Distortion Box

As we talked about in the first half of the book, a large majority of adult entertainers snared in the Trap eventually end up with a grossly distorted sense of reality and their own personal worth and identity. They start taking bigger risks and care less and less about their own personal safety.

Guess what? Viewers are not immune to the reality distortion box.

We already covered this to a lesser degree earlier with the fantasy cage and the narcissist cage. Because porn seems particularly effective at lulling audiences into a state of flow, there is a very real potential for negative cognitive consequences. The viewer's brain is rewired. Healthy connections are torn down and parted out to form the new connections where the interests of porn take top priority.

Once addiction sinks its hooks in a person, a couple things happen. As we touched on earlier, many viewers start accepting the extremes as normal and more common than are actually the case. The viewer might envision women in a new way, reduced to having only one purpose: sexual gratification. The more a viewer relies on porn, however, the smaller the payoff. The brain constantly needs something wilder, stronger, riskier to feel that rush.

This is an extremely perilous point for a viewer who has wandered too deeply into the Trap. Not only does certain disturbing content such as rape scenes not bother him anymore, and perhaps even excites him, but there is also a strong likelihood that eventually being a passive spectator won't be enough. He might foist new fetishes or fantasies on a partner. Once that runs its course or the partner finally objects, he will have to seek out new ways to get his fix. Risk-taking heightens the buzz in a way that is almost close to the original high. Some escalate to private webcamming sessions, seek sex outside of an established partnership, or start visiting strip clubs. The titillation, as always, will be fleeting as the addiction only grows hungrier. The porn addict can very easily escalate to sex addict. He is no longer addicted to passive voyeur and has shifted to an all-consuming need to perform the physical acts that excite him and cannot function when his needs go unmet.

The odds are favorable that he will get so deep into his fantasy that he will stop being careful. He could seek out increasingly hazardous highs, like trading agency escorts for street prostitutes. He may engage in sexual affairs with strangers, stop using protection, solicit sex online, start trolling social media for someone willing to trade nudes, videos, maybe even hook up. The addict holds to the false certainty that he can compartmentalize. It is his life, and what he does on his own time is separate from the world around him. It no longer matters that his choices could not only cause him harm, but also wreak terrible collateral damage to those he cares about most. In fact, it doesn't even enter into the equation.

At this stage, the once passive viewer is dangerously preoccupied with novelty and thrill-seeking while simultaneously blinded to the very precarious ledge on which he now stands. Now the viewer is so deep in the Trap, he has no idea how to make his way back to the door of the cage, not that he would want to. Reality has fundamentally shifted, and the more the fantasy world takes over, the more his behavior spirals out of control.

Some steadily retreat deeper into the fantasy alone for various reasons. Perhaps what excites them isn't readily available or is deemed criminal. Perhaps their body dysmorphic beliefs drive them further into seclusion. PDD is a strong example. What real woman would want their tiny penis? There is an entire sub-culture in adult entertainment where men pay adult entertainers to mock and shame them for having small penises.

Again, I wish I were making this up.

The viewer could swing to the opposite extreme, where he grows delusional and overconfident. He might become sexually inappropriate with females in his life, start making passes at coworkers, friends' wives, their daughters, or strangers both in person or on social media. We don't have to search far to find porn-addicted men who have crossed socially acceptable, even sacred, lines. The addict, so caught up in the fantasy, is either unlikely to see his actions as improper or simply won't care. His divergent behavior can take on many forms mental health experts could rate along a scale from mild to extreme.

Offenders might peer in windows, set up spy cameras in what should be private areas such as public restrooms, or masturbate in public places. The risk of potentially being caught adds to the excitement. Behavior can even escalate to criminal activity, since the viewer has internalized many false beliefs, such as a woman screaming and yelling "No!" really means she is turned on. Sexual partners are no longer humans. They are merely objects whose sole reason for existence are to serve the dominant party's desires.

Crossing sacred lines and breaking taboo are common tropes in porn, which an addict might then seek to act out in life. For instance, storylines featuring incest and rape have grown increasingly popular. How long until the person is no longer satisfied with the fiction?

At this moment, maybe some reading this might believe my claims have gone too far. It's true that porn doesn't automatically turn viewers into criminals, rapists, or worse. I agree. Humans are vastly complex. The formula isn't ever that simple. If it were, it would make things so much easier. Maybe promiscuity, sex addiction, or sexually inappropriate behavior is due to nature or nurture or genetics or environment. I don't have all the answers. No one does.

But I do have my own personal experiences and more than my fair share of terrifying stalkers who had convinced themselves that we were destined to be together. This has been one of the main hindrances for me when it has come to trying to work outside of porn. Every job I took, it was only a matter of time before I had some fan cornering me on the job, trying to follow me home, or making phony appointments simply for a chance to be alone with me to act out their personal fantasies. When I refused to be part of their fantasy world, they snapped. This was when the highly detailed and graphic death threats generally would start coming in.

The reality distortion box had these fans convinced that what I did on screen was what I did all day, every day, that it was what I loved, and I couldn't wait to do with them. They couldn't separate fantasy from reality and had slipped into what psychiatric professionals refer to as erotomania.

Erotomania or de Clérambault's Syndrome, is a delusional disorder in which a person mistakenly believes they are loved by someone of higher social status or by some person who is, for whatever reason, unattainable.[8] By virtue of being a delusion, the obsessed party is unaware that what they see, feel, and experience is anything but reality. This can lead to stalking behavior and striking out at anyone the person believes is standing in the way of the fictional relationship. In extreme cases, when the object of affection fails to reciprocate and fall in line with the fantasy, the subject can turn violent or even homicidal.[9]

For me, porn was a job, a Trap I couldn't escape that was damaging my body, mind, and soul. Outside of work, I had no interest in engaging in the same sort of sexual escapades fans watched online. Yet, to the fan who has lost touch with reality, they were convinced they would be happy if they could just be with me or someone like me: a sex-toy whose entire world centered on offering them every pleasure imaginable and needing nothing in return.

This said, let's get back to Joe Normal.

He has been cooped up all year because of the pandemic, trying to survive soul-crushing stress. To cope, he clicked on some free porn and fell all the way down into the reality distortion box. He follows all his favorite porn stars online, watches for everything they post, and he comments on every thread. If his favorite star responds to any comment, even politely, Joe is certain there is something more there if you read between the lines. It's way more than a nice comment. There is a secret message, a bond he has with the star that no other man has.

She is clearly flirting with him. She wants him. They are destined for each other. He can't stand to have sex with his wife anymore because she won't or can't give him what he desires. No, he needs his star and only her, and clearly, she wants him, too. She just can't come out and say it online because there would be too many other jealous men, so she is talking in some sort of code.

After all, she did like his comment, right?

A hallmark symptom of erotomania is the stalker believes he and the object of his desire share a special connection expressed through special glances, hidden signals, or some sort of mental telepathy.[10]

Translate this online, and the generic thumbs-up like or smiley face takes on a whole new meaning for the stalker.

The reality distortion box is where interest shifts to obsession. Fans can turn into stalkers or, they have such an intense need to make their fantasy a reality, they might start doing porn.

Some male porn stars actually began as avid porn fans. Eventually, they transitioned into working in adult entertainment because they couldn't rest until they crossed the line from reality into their dream world. They wanted to live the life they saw on the screen. They longed to be where they could do anything, any time, to as many hot babes as they wanted. I have worked with more than a few porn-fans-turned-porn-actors. In fact, it's so common most of us don't even raise an eyebrow.

In the midst of the COVID-19 crisis and lockdowns, this trend has risen sharply, and not only because people are desperate to put food on the table. How do we know this? Go back and look at the staggering numbers of new OnlyFans accounts or how even Pornhub boasted that "amateur" was so popular a term as to define their year in 2019, the year right before the pandemic.

Many regular everyday people are no longer content to watch porn, they want to post porn online. They want to act out what they have been watching passively and, because they are amateurs, far too many are doing this without protection, regular testing for disease or proper safety measures. Any fan who crosses that line from audience to performer will be chained by the same computer algorithms and facial recognition software that dooms all other adult entertainers. He will bear the same Scarlet XXX, because this kind of wish-fulfillment is a fast-pass to the porn box and being marked for life.

Clearly this isn't the experience of every person or couple who views porn or engages in adult entertainment, but it is the experience for enough people that it merits concern. The point is that the industry is never going to admit openly that fans can get hurt as well. Again, the industry must pretend the Trap doesn't exist.

As for Joe Normal? He is making seriously bad decisions with no concept that he is sitting on a time bomb of his own making. Either he is caught in a cycle of crippling guilt and shame, or he is now so hardened that he actually believes he isn't doing anything wrong, that he can't or won't be discovered. Any moment, he can be exposed, but he is so deeply hooked that he is blind to the very real danger. Red flags, stop signs, and stop lights have long since vanished from his line of sight. Since he has isolated himself physically or emotionally, he has lost perspective.

Joe Normal is hiding his search history, the credit card bills, or possibly even that he has stopped looking for a job or a way to reopen his business. At this point, he is in full blown denial and honestly believes he can go back to his old life any time. His relationships are either at the breaking point or already broken, but he no longer cares because he simply doesn't see it. His wife, kids, family, friends, business, finances, reputation, or even his own personal safety and freedom no longer matter. He truly believes he is still in control and not doing anything wrong.

Invincibility is a major part of the delusion.

Joe Junior isn't immune to the reality distortion box simply because he is a teenager. The *New York Times* posted an article, "We Know It Harms Kids to See Smoking on TV. What About Rape?" that offers some food for thought. Similarly, heeding the recommendation of medical experts, Netflix cut the suicide scene from the popular series *13 Reasons Why*. Following on the heels of this, Netflix has pledged to remove smoking from all upcoming original productions aimed at younger audiences. The company has also mandated smoking be included among other content warnings such as gore, violence, and strong language.[11]

If we refer to the July 4, 2019, *NPR* article, "Netflix Promises to Quit Smoking on (Most) Original Programming," by Vanessa Romo, Netflix has acted on cautions highlighted by the Truth Initiative, America's largest nonprofit organization dedicated to fighting nicotine addiction. This organization warned that what young viewers see on the small screen can have a drastic impact on their future health.[12] According to the Truth Initiative in that article:

Based on estimated viewership of these programs, results suggest that approximately 28 million young people were exposed to tobacco through television and streaming programs in these most popular shows alone. That exposure is a significant public health concern, because viewing tobacco use in on-screen entertainment media is a critical factor associated with young people starting to smoke.[13]

If depictions of smoking and suicide have been deemed so harmful to our younger generations, what about rape? Studies have demonstrated compelling evidence that young males who watched shows that depicted sexual assault and rape in commercial programming were consequently more at ease with violent acts against females and more aroused by sexually aggressive acts compared to those males who had never been exposed to such content. We are talking HBO and the like here, not porn.[14]

If companies like Netflix are concerned about young people seeing smoking, suicide, sexual aggression, and rape enough to either remove the content from all upcoming productions or rate those programs for an older audience and include specific warnings, then clearly, they take the studies showing potential harm seriously.

Given the open access children and adolescents have to even the most violent and depraved porn, we would be irresponsible to blindly accept that porn doesn't present any potentially negative or even dangerous impacts on mental wellness. If the largest health organizations are concerned that young people watching smoking as a normalized or even cool activity might make them future smokers, then doesn't the logic extend to porn? If young males watch sex in context of violence and domination, then why wouldn't we be equally troubled this content could contribute to a rising generation of abusers and rapists?

If Joe Junior has made it this far into the Trap, how this level of addiction manifests could take on any number of forms. A lot depends on Joe Junior's personality. He might isolate, cut off friendships, and abandon the activities that once fulfilled him. He no longer takes time for sports or friends because he is dedicating every free moment to porn. The opposite could happen as well. Since he is an athlete, and porn is a common sideline with teenage boys, he could bond with peers who share his new hobby. They trade sites and recommendations and get together to watch porn as if for sport. Toxic masculinity is reinforced throughout the friend group, which now resembles more of a pack. His attitude toward females degrades in lockstep with his friends' outlook. Girls and women are bitches, sluts, whores, and dehumanized disposable things.

Porn culture is wreaking havoc on high school students, both male and female. Sexting is the new flirting. Revenge porn and doxing have become major issues for teens. Cases of sexual harassment, rape, and gang rape are steadily rising. Additionally, the social media-fueled, "Boys will be boys" attitude that excuses inexcusable behavior is at an all-time high. This is yet another topic that could be its own book, so I strongly recommend the award-winning 2018 documentary, *Roll Red Roll*, in the interest of brevity.

Suffice to say Joe Junior is already living most of his life in a sexually toxic culture that is getting more and more out of control, and the pandemic has only exacerbated the problem. Who knows what the long-term impact of so many lockdowns, long periods of isolation, and increased reliance on technology for education, entertainment, and socializing will be?

Joe Junior can fall prey to rape culture, but there is a box that the Trap has uniquely crafted for young males.

The Incel Box

The incel box is an extreme variant of the reality distortion box. Incel stands for "involuntarily celibate," and is a descriptor that has been adopted by deeply misogynistic men who blame women for their inability to engage in sex, and thus, deserve punishment and retribution for this perceived slight.

Like other hate groups, incel beliefs and attitudes run along a spectrum. According to the April 25, 2018, *GQ* article by Eleanor Halls

"Who Are the 'Incels'? The Involuntary Celibates Who Want Women Punished,":

> *Incels often believe women should be verbally shamed and, in extreme, physically punished with sexual assault, rape or disfigurement. Coming together on Internet communities such as Reddit, 'incels' categorise society into two camps, the 'Chads' (attractive men) and 'femoids' or 'Stacys' (attractive women who the Chads find attractive).* [15]

Though the incel ideology splinters into many camps, their core issue is simple: sex. In the incel mind, the one thing they desire (sex) is permanently out of reach and always due to reasons beyond their control. There are incels who blame this forced celibacy on being too short. Some fixate on the small size of their wrists. Others believe it's because they don't have a large enough penis, the right jawline, etc. One could reasonably assert that incel beliefs are what happens when severe body dysmorphia and profound self-loathing combine, igniting unquenchable rage.

The article, "How Many Bones Would You Break to Get Laid? 'Incels' are going under the knife to reshape their faces, and their dating prospects," is a heart-breaking glimpse into the incel mind. Some incels have spent veritable fortunes on plastic surgery to be more appealing to females. Yet, when they do attract female attention, their hatred and revulsion only intensifies. [16] For women, it's a no-win situation.

The incel resents women forcing them to become Chads to be worthy of receiving sex. If he has surgery, the incel is the same person on the inside, thus he loathes any female who now finds him attractive because it is a clear indication of how shallow she is in the first place. It's a circular logic that cements men as hapless victims and females as enemy, oppressor, and tormentor. [17]

Why am I taking time to mention incels? Because this radical misogyny appears to be particularly appealing to young males, many of whom are then becoming increasingly radicalized by it. On September 10, 2020, the Anti-Defamation League (ADL) posted unsettling findings in its report, "Online Poll Results Provide New Insights into Incel Community,":

> *In March 2020, moderators at incel.co, one of the largest incel online forums, released the results of a community poll. Incels are generally perceived/believed to be young, white men. The March 2020 poll results largely confirm that profile: 82 percent of respondents said they were between the ages of 18 and 30. The largest percentage (36 percent) were between the ages of 18 and 21. The second largest segment (27.9 percent) said they were between 22 and 25, followed by 18.1 percent aged 26-30. Perhaps most alarmingly, nearly 8 percent said they were younger than 17.*[18]

Though it deeply saddens me that anyone would fall prey to hate ideology, what stood out to me was that almost eight percent of incels were under the age of seventeen. Keep in mind that this poll hardly provides real numbers since only those incels willing to take the poll offer us any data. How many remained silent? A poll like this can only, at best, reveal a shadowy outline of larger forces. Yet, while polls and surveys might reveal the blurry form of a larger crisis, the sharp rise in incel attacks over the past seven years that have left fifty-three people dead and scores injured paints a chilling picture.[19]

On May 23, 2014, twenty-two-year-old Elliot Rodger killed six people and injured fourteen others before finally taking his own life. Rodger identified as an incel in the now infamous one hundred thirty-seven-page autobiography, "My Twisted World, The Story of Elliot Rodger," released in *The New York Times*.[20] Rodger's manifesto underscores many of the disruptive social shifts threaded throughout this book. Instead of interacting with peers in person, Rodger steadily withdrew into the online world, a place he could control. He could only connect with others via chat and message boards, and eventually, his life revolved around hiding in the virtual reality of online gaming.[21]

Though Rodger is hardly a reliable narrator when it comes to objective analysis, his skewed self-perception may sadly be the most revealing and valuable set of observations. His autobiography pinpoints specific events that he believed changed/doomed him. For instance, in sixth grade, he claimed that while chatting online another member of the group sent him an unsolicited stream of nude pictures of women. He noted how his body reacted in a way that simultaneously fascinated and terrified him, much like we see in chapter 12 with the negative psychological consequences for children, particularly young males, being exposed to porn.[22]

Though Rodger admits he was never comfortable with girls, he claims his severe anxiety and deepening resentment toward females began when he first witnessed them as objects of lust. At thirteen, an older teen introduced him to pornographic movies. Seeing women in the context of sex only added fuel to the proverbial fire. He confessed to watching porn and being unable to stop masturbating. Riddled with shame, guilt, and crushing low self-esteem, he only continued to retreat inward, isolate, and look to porn as a substitute for venturing out and interacting with the opposite sex in person.[23]

In the end, it appears that weighed down under unrealistic images in mass media, pop culture, and supernormal stereotypes in porn, Rodger fell into a death-spiral of self-loathing and hate that ultimately ended in tragedy.

Though Elliot Rodger is an extreme example, various studies reveal seriously disturbing trends. Not only are incel groups getting larger, but they appear to be radicalizing at an astonishing pace. According to an article in the *MIT Technology Review*, "The 'manosphere' is getting more toxic as angry men join the incels," the incel threat level has increased to the degree that top computer scientists have joined forces to study how and why this group is swiftly radicalizing as well as what part technology plays in this paradigm shift.[24] The article references the study "The Evolution of the Manosphere Across the Web"[25] and offers only a slice of the overall bleak picture the data is revealing:

> *The team's analysis found that the manosphere is evolving—and fast.*
> *Over the past 10 years, the population of men identifying as men's rights*

activists and MGTOW (Men Going Their Own Way)—traditionally older and less violent—is falling while younger, more toxic PUA (Pick Up Artists) and incel communities have seen a spike.

Worryingly, it seems that there has been a significant migration from men's rights groups to incel groups. Every year since 2015, around 8% of MRA (Men's Rights Activists) or MGTOW members appear to have become more radicalized and joined incel groups online.[26]

In January of 2020, the Texas Department of Public Safety released a report that specifically listed incels as, "an emerging domestic terrorism threat as current adherents demonstrate marked acts or threats of violence in furtherance of their social grievance."[27]

Is online porn creating incels, and in particular, violent incels? Again, there are no simple answers or straight lines. While there is much we don't know, there is much we can intelligently deduce with the facts we do have. We know that especially with the COVID-19 pandemic and lockdowns, people are isolated and forced to interact mainly online or settle for being alone. With more and more of the global population either being forced into isolation or pressured into self-isolation to combat a virus, it's hard not to worry about the long-term psychological impact.

Online socialization simply cannot replace hundreds of thousands of years of human experience and developmental requisites.

While virtual reality is not reality, given enough time and exposure, the mind has a harder and harder time distinguishing between the two. The supernormal overwrites the normal and wreaks havoc on body image, self-esteem, relationships, and mental health.

The Thing About Boxes

No viewer deserves the hells that await in these boxes. In fact, I don't like the idea of anyone in a box. I have been put in a box most of my life, and it is a terrible place to get stuck. Alas, that is the Trap's end goal. So long as adult entertainers can never really leave the industry, the Trap grows larger and hungrier. Even if a porn actress does somehow wriggle free of the porn box, her videos and content will remain up and available long after she has aged out, burned out, or bled out.

Porn stars can't even die with dignity. Trolls fill their social media and web pages with hate and spite even after the girl is long in the grave.

While entertainers are almost, by default, condemned to eternity in a box, the same can't be said about porn viewers. Ideally, our society will learn to have compassion, offer grace, and give performers the opportunity to live a new and better life. Perhaps this book is a step in that direction. One can dream, right?

Unless our society makes some major changes, performers are almost doomed to an eternal sentence in the Trap as soon as they set foot beyond the door. Their content can long outlive them, and they can never, ever be forgotten.

Porn viewers must be wary as well. Life as a spectator isn't nearly as safe as the Trap wants its audience to believe. The porn industry can claim all it wants that it isn't addictive, but then they have a lot of explaining to do when it comes to the stats. The math simply doesn't compute.

According to Pornhub's very own press page, the site is (as of end of 2020):

One of the most prolific adult websites, averaging over 100 billion video views a year, roughly 12.5 porn videos per person on Earth. Pornhub enjoys over 100 million visits a day, over 36 billion visits per year, and over 125 million daily visits to the Pornhub Network of sites including YouPorn and Redtube. There are currently 20 million registered Pornhub users. Average streaming bandwidth of 120 Gigabytes per second. Average visit duration of 9 minutes and 59 seconds. 74% of Pornhub visitors are men, 26% are women. Average age of Pornhub users is 35.3 years, with 60% being under the age of 35. 76% of traffic comes from mobile devices including smartphones and tablets. [Emphasis added][28]

If we only break down the number of registered users, 12 million viewers out of 20 million are the millennial generation and younger, and the Pornhub family of sites only represent a portion of all the sites providing adult content. Given all the scientific studies, the research, and data, the Trap is molding the hearts, minds, and beliefs of those who hold our future in their hands.

18

NO MORE DEAD MEAT

When I originally outlined the book and named the chapters, I had planned on this chapter mirroring the same one in the first half of the book. Chapter 9's "Meet Ms. Meat" was to have a counterpart: "Meet Mr. Dead Meat." The symmetry was appealing. But, when I reached the end of chapter 17, I had an epiphany. This book didn't require a specific chapter to meet Mr. Dead Meat because we are already well-acquainted by this point.

Once a casual porn viewer slips over into addiction, he has taken an exit ramp off a main thoroughfare and been rerouted into a vast nexus of highways with no speed limits, no rules, and no danger signs. So caught up in the wild ride, the addict has no idea that all such highways lead to any number of personal hells as unique as his fingerprints.

This last part of the Trap is for the condemned who have no way out. Brick by brick, many addicts have been building walls around themselves. The walls that have become their cells and, ultimately, self-made tombs. The false sense of invincibility catches up and costs them everything. This is the point of no return. There is no reversing an HIV diagnosis, a prison sentence, or a scandal that forever links their name with disgrace or infamy.

It is time we take a stand.

What exactly are we standing against? I can already hear the protests: *People need to lighten up. Sex isn't bad. If we were just more comfortable with our sexuality, porn wouldn't be a problem. Our culture is too uptight.*

If our society ever becomes evolved enough that brutal gang bangs, incest, kidnapping, torture, and sex with children is considered progress, is that a really society we want to be a part of? That is a question we need to ask.

How can we cry out for gender equality, denounce toxic masculinity, and demand an end to sexual assault while simultaneously accepting the messages commonly portrayed in online porn, where sex, humiliation, domination, and violence so frequently go together? How can we claim we love and value our children when online porn sites push content featuring "barely legal" girls and boys, or worse?

While many viewers might assume that the actors are of legal age, recently it's come to light that many of the videos that Pornhub featured were actually minors. This is why Pornhub had to jettison a massive portion of their content or face the legal consequences.

According to Nicholas Kristof's December 4, 2020, exposé in the *New York Times*, "The Children of Pornhub,":

> *Its (Pornhub's) site is infested with rape videos. It monetizes child rapes, revenge pornography, spy cam videos of women showering, racist and misogynist content, and footage of women being asphyxiated in plastic bags. A search for 'girls under18' (no space) or '14yo' leads in each case to more than 100,000 videos. Most aren't of children being assaulted, but too many are.*
>
> *...Pornhub profited this fall from a video of a naked woman being tortured by a gang of men in China. It is monetizing video compilations with titles like 'Screaming Teen,' 'Degraded Teen' and 'Extreme Choking.' Look at a choking video and it may suggest also searching for 'She Can't Breathe.'*[1]

I understand this has probably been a tough book to read. Trust me, it has been a tough one to write. But this is crucial foundational information and context that we need to know in order to have real conversations about how to reverse the damage effectively and set a course for a better and brighter tomorrow.

There are so many issues in the world that we can't change. We can't stop war, disease, death, natural disasters, etc. But the Trap? We can stop the Trap. We can rip it up by its roots. After this *New York Times* exposé, Pornhub found itself in the hot seat. They took down a massive chunk of content and changed who was allowed to upload content. The company even made it where the content was no longer downloadable. Or at least, it's what they have promised. Time will tell.

While this is great, how many of those videos have been up for months and years and downloaded hundreds of millions of times all over the world? Maybe Pornhub and its sister sites will get and keep their act together, but the content is out there. It is only a matter of time before it surfaces again and again. But more worryingly, why did it take a *New York Times* article to make the company suddenly realize it had a certain degree of social and moral responsibility?

19

SHUTTING DOWN THE TRAP

As I have already stated, the Trap is a foreign entity, an invasive species that is only growing larger, stronger, and hungrier. Powered by amoral algorithms, the Trap has one objective: profit at any cost.

That mathematical profit, however, is coming at the expense of real flesh and blood humans. The Trap doesn't care that an adult entertainer can never be forgotten, never start over, never truly leave the industry. The Trap doesn't bother with trivialities like ensuring what is caught on film is consensual and the parties involved are of legal age. No, the Trap relies on the audience's loneliness and ignorance, because without these, it might cease to exist. Viewers assume what they see is consensual and legal. So long as no one asks too many tough questions, the Trap lets people keep assuming. No need for any due diligence unless someone raises too much of a fuss.

By the same token, the Trap doesn't care about the long-term effects of their content. Quite the contrary. Porn is healthy and can add a fresh spark to your marriage or partnership. Sure. Nothing like hundreds of thousands of rape scenarios to cement a loving relationship. While we can't have smoking scenes in Netflix movies lest kids pick up a pack a day habit, unsupervised children and teens watching hundreds of hours of torture porn is totally fine.

The Trap doesn't check identification, doesn't care if it hooks a nine-year-old or a thirty-nine-year-old, so long as the ad money keeps flowing. It isn't the porn sites' problem that kids lie. Parents and guardians should have set up better blocks on their internet and been paying more attention to their children.

Can you imagine any other business being allowed to operate this freely and without consequence? I can't. There comes a time where we must draw a line and hold these companies accountable. It isn't as if we haven't done it before. Just try to remember the last time you saw a Joe Camel ad on television. We do have the power to stop the Trap from enjoying unregulated, unchecked freedom to do as it pleases.

Most of this book has been dedicated to education because that's always the first step in solving any problem. I have spent most of my life stuck in the Trap and have lost count how many times I almost gave up all hope.

I don't have all the solutions, but I do have a few ideas. Maybe I can use the bad things that happened to me for good. The following aren't all the answers and might not even be the best answers, but we have to start somewhere.

Hold Corporations, Executives, and Programmers Accountable

Corporations hide behind the excuse that their self-evolving algorithms are amoral, thus cannot discern the difference between right and wrong. According to them, the algorithms have one job: keep a viewer watching as long as possible to maximize the number of ad impressions. It isn't their fault Joe Normal began watching college coeds and that the self-evolving algorithms progressively nudged him over to gang rape videos.

The algorithms don't have a conscience. They simply suggested content their customer might like. The programming performed an analysis and made an educated guess based on Joe Normal's other online behaviors and scraps of collated data that he had left laying around on the internet. No one forced him to click and keep clicking on steadily more violent porn. That's all free will, baby.

Or is it?

Tristan Harris began his career working at Google. He is now a tech insider currently pioneering ethical design. He originally became concerned when it became overwhelmingly clear to him that the primary goal of Google's email design was to make it increasingly addictive. He made a statement in the documentary *The Social Dilemma* that was not only particularly poignant, but also highly relevant to my assertions:

> *"We were so concerned about that point when technology would surpass human strengths, we didn't consider at what point it would surpass human weakness."*[1]

It doesn't take much for an algorithm to nudge us toward our baser natures which are governed by the most primitive parts of our brains, the lizard brain that we discussed earlier. It's easy for the algorithms to do this because the lizard brain is particularly vulnerable to manipulation.

Software executives, designers, programmers, and engineers all know this. They count on it, actually. They use our lizard brains against us, knowing that we will naturally gravitate to supernormal stimuli and seek out novelty. It is simply how we are wired. Corporations have deconstructed our biological imperatives then used that knowledge to alter our behavior to fulfill their goal: profit.

So, one possible solution is for us to demand ethical design. Unlimited economic incentive, shareholder pressure, and allowing businesses to self-regulate is a toxic formula for this sort of corrosive business model. Whether we like it or not, it is up to us to hold these companies accountable.

If an algorithm or a program doesn't have a "conscience," whose fault is that? While algorithms, software, and computers might not have an innate moral compass, those who create the code do, or at least they should. Last I checked, humans own and operate the companies and direct the business and programming initiatives. Humans manage these departments and set the objectives for the engineers, developers and designers who write the software. Humans program the algorithms and can change the parameters of those algorithms to something better than profit at any price. They can, but so far, they haven't had to.

Up until this point, we have largely allowed the online porn industry, like many other tech giants, to govern themselves. They have been allowed to put profit ahead of people. Unless there is a financial or legal reason to change, why would they? If we want them to act more responsibly, then we have to hit them where it will hurt: the bottom line.

One of the main reasons I spent so much time explaining the surveillance capitalism model is because understanding how this system generates such staggering profit offers us ways to rein in the online porn monstrosity without resorting to flat-out censorship.

Data Tax

For instance, we could tax the amount of data collection and processing much the same way a power company would charge per kilowatt hour of use. Any company that specializes in gathering every shred of digital activity for the purposes of generating behavioral predictive models would no longer be able to mine our everyday human experiences for free.

Think about mineral rights and the Barnett Shale natural gas boom in Texas and parts of Oklahoma and surrounding states. For many years, whenever someone bought a home or property, the deed also included mineral rights as part of the deal. Thus, when the gas companies finally came up with technology capable of extracting the natural gas from beneath the Barnett Shale, one of the largest onshore natural gas fields, they couldn't simply drill anywhere they wanted for free. Not legally, anyway.[2] The gas companies had to negotiate with the property owner first to get permission even to drill.

Landowners had a choice and an option to say no. Landowners who agreed to allow the gas companies to set up a well also negotiated proper compensation.

Our online behaviors are valuable. We are a natural resource that companies want to tap into, refine, then sell in a global marketplace to outside parties. The difference, however, is that these companies are often doing this without our knowledge or consent. They are the ones making unprecedented profits, even though they are selling our lives.

As long as these corporations are allowed to siphon up every atom of information available at no cost to them, there is no reason to change how they do business. But if suddenly they had to pay taxes on their data collection, this might at least deter them from hoovering up every nugget of data on the planet. They could still data mine, just not for free. This new source of tax revenue could be repurposed to combat child pornography, shut down human trafficking, or go to helping victims of rape, abuse, domestic violence, and exploitation.

Advertising Transparency

We have discussed how it is possible for online porn to be free and the fact that it really isn't free at all. Large companies are essentially underwriting the operation knowing that they will have a guaranteed, captive audience who will see their ads. Using the data collection and algorithmic profiles, these companies know which viewers to target with what product. It is an efficient advertising model, but consumers have a right to know what their buying power is supporting.

We already do something similar in the diamond market. There are sound reasons for purchasing diamonds from reputable jewelers. A jeweler can make sure the diamond the customer is purchasing has been ethically sourced and is not a "blood diamond." Blood diamonds, also called "conflict diamonds," are most often mined using slave labor in war-torn countries and the profits fund military insurgents.[3]

If big brands who profit from advertising on internet porn sites were legally required to list how and where they advertise, say, in an annual report, they might decide that publicly linking their name with porn just isn't the direction they want their brand to go. More likely, consumers and investors would make that choice for them, and shouldn't that be our prerogative? Shouldn't consumers know if they are supporting a brand that markets on porn sites? Particularly sites that have little to no content oversight and few if any barriers to stop minors from gaining access?

Shareholders obviously want the highest returns possible, but at what cost? Sure, everyone wants a nice retirement, but I imagine they would also like to be able to sleep at night, too. If brands knew fund managers were watching with a sharper eye, they might be pickier about which sites they partnered with or use their influence to make sure any adult sites they did advertise on eradicated illegal content, added extra moderators, and put in extra safeguards to prevent minors from gaining entry.

Advertising & Marketing Restrictions

Alcohol and tobacco companies already have insanely strict guidelines as to where and how they can advertise. These industries cannot market in any way or on any medium that influences minors. If a company that doesn't sell age-restricted products, such as cologne or designer clothing, wants to market on porn sites, then why shouldn't that company be legally required to choose their target demographic? Adults or children, which is it?

If their product is something that is marketed to adults as well as minors, then why should they be allowed to have the best of all worlds? They shouldn't. If a company wants to advertise a body wash, vitamin supplement, or new social media platform on porn sites, then fine, but that's it. All other marketing venues are then forfeit. By advertising on porn sites, they have then chosen to only advertise to an adult market. They don't get to straddle both worlds. Cigarette companies don't get to, so why should other brands be held to a different standard?

Alcohol and tobacco companies are also legally prohibited from marketing in ways that could entice young children, yet porn pop-up ads seem to sprout up everywhere. Joe Camel was a hard "no," because he was a cartoon that essentially was grooming underage kids to become future smokers. All right, but what about all these porn pop-up ads with glitter, sparkles and boobs? It seems more than a bit hypocritical. Shouldn't adult sites be held to the same advertising restrictions as other products off-limits to minors?

Looks like a no-brainer to me.

Regulate FREE Porn

By now, I feel I have made it pretty clear that porn has plenty of downfalls and negative consequences. Despite all the potential harm porn can do, I suffer no illusions that adult entertainment will go away. I believe if we tried to completely ban porn, the cure would be far worse than the disease.

It would only drive the market deeper underground, where those who are already being victimized would only suffer more. Censorship would only shift offenders even further beyond the reach of law enforcement. It's a nightmare scenario. The slippery slope of censorship and what it can do to a society is too dangerous to even tread this direction. The cure can't be worse than the disease, so to speak.

While I don't believe banning porn would be even remotely effective, web hosting companies can refuse to do business with sites dedicated to serving up the most extreme and violent varieties of porn. If the more popular adult entertainment sites vet videos more thoroughly, it might at the least remove the more reprehensible and borderline or outright criminal content from mainstream sites and relegate the extreme porn to fringe sites. Sure, the most heinous material would probably find a nice shadowy corner on the dark web or open up shop in countries with little-to-no regulation, but at least their dangerous content wouldn't be normalized by virtue of being included with content that mainstream companies offer. It might also make it easier for law enforcement to shut them down since their videos aren't intermingled with hundreds of millions of pieces of legitimate content.

Mainstream companies like Pornhub have used protections afforded by Section 230 of the Communications Decency Act to escape responsibility. There is no reason this protection can't be defined and circumscribed in ways that force these sites to improve self-policing or suffer consequences.

Pornhub is already mending its ways, but consumers need to keep up the pressure and make sure the company holds to what it's promised. Modern audiences have a short attention span, so will Pornhub still have the same safeguards in a year, in two years, in three years? I hope so, but if we hope to enjoy any kind of lasting changes the public needs to remain vigilant and vocal, as do advertisers and investors. If Pornhub and other sites don't keep their word, the audience is in the best position to keep them accountable. Never underestimate the power of public pressure. Demand better. My goal with this book has been to shine a light in the darkness, to let the everyday person see the truth then make an informed decision on whether the high price of free is really worth it.

End Occupational Discrimination

We are now looping back to where we began, to the performers. We have to allow them a way out of the Trap. Especially now that the industry is digitizing movies that are decades old, should a person who made a decision as a teen or a young person be made to pay forever for what society still sees as a moral transgression? How long is it until someone can be forgiven for work that was/is legal? Because, as it stands, we have entire generations from millennials going back to baby boomers who could possibly be outed. Not to mention the future impact on the lives of everyday people who were simply trying to survive during COVID-19. That's a lot of judgement and why? For what? Is the punishment really fitting the crime?

On January 19, 2021, Marlow Stern at *The Daily Beast* broke a story, "She was Fired from Taco Bell for Being in Porn."[4] Sex worker Lonna Wells, concerned about the pandemic, put her career in adult entertainment on hold and took a job at the fast-food chain Taco Bell to provide for her family in the meantime. Wells was forthright about her history as a sex worker, and the manager claimed that would not be a problem. Yet, after less than a week on the job, she received a phone call telling her that her employment had been terminated. When she asked why, she received the answer that, "...a customer had lodged a formal complaint that there was a woman working the drive-thru who was doing internet porn, and as a God-fearing Christian they didn't feel comfortable giving the establishment their business."[5]

My first question is, "How would a God-fearing Christian recognize a porn star in the first place?" My second question is, "Where's a good smiting when you need one?"

Ironically, Lonna Wells, raised in a Christian Pentecostal home, was crushed knowing a stranger used had Christianity as a reason to have her fired. She is even quoted as saying, "One of the first things I was taught was that you're not supposed to judge others—only God is supposed to do that."[6]

Christian "charity" aside, Lonna Wells can't count on any support from the legal system either. According to the Arkansas Department of Labor and Licensing:

> *Arkansas recognizes the doctrine of 'employment at will.' This means that, as a general rule, either the employer or the employee may end the employment relationship at any time for any reason or for no reason at all. There are, however, a number of exceptions to this general rule under state and federal law. For example, state and federal law prohibit an employer from firing an employee on the basis of age, sex, race, religion, national origin, disability or genetic information. Also, a woman cannot be fired because she is pregnant or has had an abortion.*[7]

Arkansas can justify what happened to Wells using legal gymnastics. The state considers it, "[...]a crime to perform sexual acts in exchange for compensation," thereby outlawing all consensual sex work. At what point was Lonna Wells charged, tried and convicted in the state of Arkansas or any other state? What if she didn't even make films in Arkansas and legally filmed in Los Angeles? It doesn't matter. Like so many others, Wells has no recourse and no options except to return to sex work.

Until we put an end to occupational and societal discrimination, anyone who ends up in adult entertainment or porn either willingly or unwillingly can never leave.

Of course, once this article was published, Taco Bell's corporate office released an official statement, and *The Daily Beast* article was amended with this update:

> *Taco Bell team members come from diverse backgrounds and experiences and all are welcome into the Taco Bell family. This former team member worked for a franchise location and the franchisee has informed us that the accusations made are not accurate and that she was instead terminated for violation of their policies and procedures.* [8]

Lonna Wells violated policies and procedures. How amazingly vague and incredibly convenient! Wells was only taking a break from adult entertainment, but the message seems fairly clear. If she can't even take a break, odds are she can't ever retire either.

We have become a culture that permits tech giants to hide behind Section 230 protections while profiting off rape, child porn, revenge porn, and spycam footage featuring everyday women and girls in bathrooms, dressing rooms and other private places. Worse than that, we have become a culture that rewards them.

According to that same article in the *New York Times*, "The Children of Pornhub,":

> *Pornhub is owned by MindGeek, a private pornography conglomerate with more than 100 websites, production companies and brands. Its sites*

include Redtube, YouPorn, Xtube, Spankwire, Extremetube, Men.Com, MyDirtyHobby, Thumbzilla, PornMD, Brazzers and GayTube. There are other major players in porn outside the Mindgeek umbrella, most notably xHamster and XVIDEOS, but Mindgeek is a porn titan. If it operated in another industry, the Justice Department could be discussing an antitrust case against it.

Pornhub and Mindgeek also stand out because of their influence. One study this year by a digital marketing company concluded that Pornhub was the technology company with the third greatest-impact on society in the 21st century, after Facebook and Google but ahead of Microsoft, Apple and Amazon.[9]

When called to account for profiting off pain, these tech giants wail that they just don't have enough moderators to properly vet every single video uploaded. The internet is too big, too complex to keep little kids from accessing adult content. So they remain in business because they promise to do better.

Oh, okay. Good enough for me.

Or not.

Mindgeek is a private company owned by Feras Antoon, David Marmorstein Tasillo, and Bernard Bergemar. As owners of a technology company estimated to have the third greatest impact on the twenty-first century, I think it's safe to say these guys aren't in need of a side job at Taco Bell to keep the lights on, even after purging a large portion of their content.

Advertisers, as we have already mentioned, also make fortunes targeting online porn audiences, even those viewers not yet old enough to watch a PG-13 movie. Companies revel in record profits marketing on the same platforms that have rendered women like Lonna Wells, Resa Woodward, Kirsten Vaughn, and countless others unemployable and banished from polite society forever.

Am I the only one seeing a problem here?

20

LOVE UNLOCKS THE TRAP

W ell, we made it. I hope you see the adult entertainment and porn industry with new eyes and from many perspectives. Everyone on both sides of the screen has a story. All of us carry around our own bit of brokenness.

We no longer live in the same world as our parents and their Leave-it-to-Beaver idylls. Technology long ago outpaced our brains, legal systems, values, and expectations. It is as if the internet is a giant magnet that has set our moral compasses spinning wildly, unable to locate true north and find our bearings.

In these final pages, I would like you to set aside porn for a moment and simply think about your life.

Have you ever said something horrible? In a moment of weakness, have you done something reckless? Have you ever made a joke that hurt the other person deeply instead of making them laugh? Have you ever done or said anything that you would give everything to take back? To do over? To make a different choice or take a different path?

Have you ever made a decision that, at the time, seemed like a good idea, only it turned out to be a disaster? Have you ever been faced with only a handful of choices, none of them good? You had to simply pick the best of the worst and pray it worked out in the end. Have you ever done your best, only to end up stuck with the consequences of other people's bad decisions?

I would wager most of you reading would say yes to most or all of the above.

Before the internet, our mistakes, missteps, addictions, and outbursts weren't permanently preserved so that we could be judged for all time. Yet, our young people are growing up terrified of life, and for good reasons. Every screwup is recorded in permanent digital ink on a permanent digital record that anyone anywhere can access at any time, even into the future. A thoughtless tweet, a brash comment, a picture no one else was supposed to see? They can all change a life in an instant or end a future at the speed of Fios.

Those who are old enough to remember life before the digital age, would you have taken the risks, made the mistakes, broken new ground if you worried that every bad choice you made would be used against you in the court of public opinion for as long as you lived and longer?

Envision the worst moments of your life. Time heals all wounds, right? You got too drunk at a party, thought you were in love and had no idea the person was filming, or maybe you were only a kid and had no idea what was happening. Perhaps you once did drugs, got addicted to pills, cheated on your partner, struggled with alcohol, cut corners on your taxes, or lost your temper and acted like a raving lunatic at your job. Now put these lowest moments of your life on video to be uploaded over and over no matter how many times you fight to have them taken down. Hell's whack-a-mole, indeed.

Months or years go by, and you find new places to live, new jobs, new friends. People seem to like you, then the whispering starts. You keep losing jobs for vague, flimsy reasons. Time after time, you believe you have found love, but it's only a matter of time until the light in their eyes just winks out because they no longer see you anymore; they only see the video.

There is no redemption, no future, no do-overs. Is this a world you want to live in, that you would want for your children, or for your grandchildren? Because here we are again. Our species is in check. Whether or not it's a checkmate...

Your move.

ABOUT THE AUTHOR

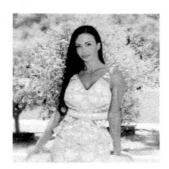

Jewels Jade is a nice Catholic girl from San Diego. She has a nursing degree, a real estate license, a Navy Seal husband, two kids, a Penthouse Pet title, and more than 500 adult films to her name.

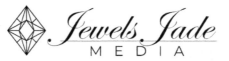

facebook.com/jewelsjademedia
twitter.com/jewelsjademedia
instagram.com/jewelsjademedia

ACKNOWLEDGMENTS

If this book is the funhouse mirror of the adult entertainment industry, then writing it has been the biggest, baddest rollercoaster ride of my life. I could not have done this without the boundless encouragement of my fans and the tireless support of my editorial team and family.

First, I would like to thank my agent, Mark Lewis, for giving me the grace of taking me seriously when I told him about this project. Your enthusiasm and excitement gave me the boost I needed not only to get over the finish line, but also to have the courage to say the things that really matter.

As I said in the first chapter, I dreamed of writing this book for fifteen years, and if it hadn't been for Kristen Lamb, it might have been another fifteen years before I even tried to write it. Coach, concept editor, and writing guru extraordinaire, Kristen not only taught me how to find the right words, but also how to find the words when I had none for things that were too difficult or painful to write. Her insight, ideas, and relentless pursuit of "the end" is what made this book possible.

But a first draft is only a draft. It took the expert editing of self-proclaimed "picky b*tch" Cait Reynolds to make the copy shine. It's not just that she knows her grammar. She can critique arguments, work magic with pacing and flow, and polish copy until it's the best it can be while staying true to the author's voice.

But wait, there's more! Once the manuscript is done, it still needs to get out into the world, and that is where the fabulous Gen Stutz comes in. Not only did she format the Kindle and paperback editions, but she masterminded how to position the book on Amazon for maximum impact. She says it's just knowing how keywords and algorithms work, but I'm pretty sure there's some black ops involved, and she's simply not saying.

Finally, I want to thank my husband of twenty years. He has stayed by my side through all the ups and downs of trying to build a career in this industry. Without him, I would not have made it out alive. He has loved me and always encouraged me to be my best self, even when all I could feel was my worst self. Through him, I have learned that love really does unlock all cages and that the truth shall set us free.

NOTES

1. Let us "Prey"

1. "The 2019 Year in Review," Pornhub Insights (Pornhub, December 11, 2019), https://www.pornhub.com/insights/2019-year-in-review.
2. Ibid.
3. Becky Little, "When Cigarette Companies Used Doctors to Push Smoking," History.com (A&E Television Networks, September 13, 2018), https://www.history.com/news/cigarette-ads-doctors-smoking-endorsement.
4. "History of the Surgeon General's Report on Smoking and Health," Centers for Disease Control and Prevention (Centers for Disease Control and Prevention, November 15, 2019), https://www.cdc.gov/tobacco/data_statistics/sgr/history/index.htm.
5. "Advertising and Promotion," Center for Tobacco Products (U.S. Food and Drug Administration, n.d.), https://www.fda.gov/tobacco-products/products-guidance-regulations/advertising-and-promotion.

2. The Bait

1. "Advertising and Promotion." Center for Tobacco Products.
2. Sam Wolfson, "Snapchat Photo Filters Linked to Rise in Cosmetic Surgery Requests," The Guardian (Guardian News and Media, August 9, 2018), https://www.theguardian.com/technology/2018/aug/08/snapchat-surgery-doctors-report-rise-in-patient-requests-to-look-filtered.

4. The Closing Door

1. "2018 Year in Review," Pornhub Insights (Pornhub, December 11, 2018), https://www.pornhub.com/insights/2018-year-in-review.
2. Ibid.
3. Ibid.
4. Ibid.
5. "The 2019 Year in Review," Pornhub Insights (Pornhub, December 11, 2019), https://www.pornhub.com/insights/2019-year-in-review.
6. Ibid.
7. Ibid.
8. Ibid.
9. Ibid.

10. Jazmin Goodwin, "Mastercard, Visa and Discover Cut Ties with Pornhub Following Allegations of Child Abuse," CNN (Cable News Network, December 14, 2020), https://www.cnn.com/2020/12/14/business/mastercard-visa-discover-pornhub/index.html.

11. "Pornhub Sets Standard for Safety and Security Policies Across Tech and Social Media; Announces Industry-Leading Measures for Verification, Moderation and Detection," Pornhub Porn Videos (Pornhub, February 2, 2021), https://www.pornhub.com/press/show?id=2172.

12. Blake Montgomery, "OnlyFans Reporting 3.5 Million New Signups in March, 60,000 of Them New Creators, per an Email from the Company. In the First Two Weeks of March Alone That Was a 75% Increase from the Normal Level.," Twitter (Twitter, March 31, 2020), https://twitter.com/blakersdozen/status/1245072167689060353?lang=en.

13. Downs, "Selling Nudes?"

14. "What Is 'SESTA/FOSTA'?" Hacking//Hustling (Hacking//Hustling, November 22, 2020), https://hackinghustling.org/what-is-sesta-fosta/.

15. Mike Masnick, "Police Realizing That SESTA/FOSTA Made Their Jobs Harder; Sex Traffickers Realizing It's Made Their Job Easier," Techdirt, May 14, 2018, https://www.techdirt.com/articles/20180509/13450339810/police-realizing-that-sesta-fosta-made-their-jobs-harder-sex-traffickers-realizing-made-their-job-easier.shtml.

16. Ibid.

17. Ewan Palmer, Billy Binion, and James R. Copland, "Sex Workers Say the Online Market Is Saturated with Performers and Fans Are Canceling Subscriptions during Coronavirus Pandemic," Newsweek, April 17, 2020, https://www.newsweek.com/coronavirus-sex-workers-cam-girls-online-1498024.

18. "Disaster Loan Assistance," SBA, n.d., https://covid19relief.sba.gov/.

19. Gabrielle Drolet and Shane O'Neill, "The Year Sex Work Came Home," The New York Times (The New York Times, April 10, 2020), https://www.nytimes.com/2020/04/10/style/camsoda-onlyfans-streaming-sex-coronavirus.html.

20. Ben Perrin, "Hope Barden: Sex Role-Play Death Prompts Law Change Plea," BBC News (BBC, July 6, 2019), https://www.bbc.com/news/uk-england-stoke-staffordshire-48790961.

21. Ibid.

22. Annie Brown, "Scots Women Warned Sex Webcamming Is Not Easy Way to Make Money during Lockdown," Daily Record (The Daily Record and Sunday Mail, May 7, 2020), https://www.dailyrecord.co.uk/news/scottish-news/women-turning-sex-webcamming-make-21993210.

23. Ibid.

5. The Lock

1. "Dissociative Disorders," NAMI, n.d., https://www.nami.org/About-Mental-Illness/Mental-Health-Conditions/Dissociative-Disorders.

2. "Xanax Addiction and Abuse - Addiction to Alprazolam," Addiction Center (Addiction Center, March 25, 2021), https://www.addictioncenter.com/benzodi-azepines/xanax/.

6. The Cage

1. "Heidi Fleiss," Wikipedia, 2021. En.Wikipedia.Org. https://en.wikipedia.org/wiki/Heidi_Fleiss.
2. Ibid.
3. Ibid.
4. Laura Italiano, "Prostitute Finally Gets Justice in Rape," New York Post (New York Post, April 16, 2010), https://nypost.com/2010/04/16/prostitute-finally-gets-justice-in-rape/.
5. "Long Island Serial Killer," Wikipedia (Wikimedia Foundation, May 20, 2021), https://en.wikipedia.org/wiki/Long_Island_serial_killer.
6. Ibid.
7. "Human Trafficking," The United States Department of Justice, November 9, 2018, https://www.justice.gov/humantrafficking.

7. The Chains that Bind

1. Eva-Marie Ayala, "Dallas Teacher's Past as Porn Actress Led to Her Firing, She Says," Dallas News (The Dallas Morning News, August 25, 2019), https://www.-dallasnews.com/news/education/2017/02/01/dallas-teacher-s-past-as-porn-actress-led-to-her-firing-she-says/.
2. Ibid.
3. Ibid.
4. Ibid.
5. Ibid.
6. Thomas Germain, "How a Photo's Hidden 'Exif' Data Exposes Your Personal Information," Consumer Reports, December 6, 2019, https://www.consumerre-ports.org/privacy/what-can-you-tell-from-photo-exif-data/.
7. Andrew Oh-Willeke, "Court: Firing Woman Due to Prior Porn Shoot Legal," The Colorado Independent, May 17, 2007, https://www.coloradoindependent.-com/2007/05/17/court-firing-woman-due-to-prior-porn-shoot-legal/.
8. "The 2019 Year in Review," Pornhub Insights.
9. Downs, "Selling Nudes?"
10. Otillia Steadman, "Her Colleagues Watched Her OnlyFans Account at Work. When Bosses Found Out, They Fired Her.," BuzzFeed News (BuzzFeed News, September 29, 2020), https://www.buzzfeednews.com/article/otilliastead-man/mechanic-fired-onlyfans-account-indiana
11. Ibid.
12. Ibid.

13. "Pornography Addiction," Sergen's Medical Dictionary (Farlex, 2012), https://medical-dictionary.thefreedictionary.com/Pornography+addiction.

14. "Internet Pornography by the Numbers," Webroot (An Opentext Company, n.d.), https://www.webroot.com/us/en/resources/tips-articles/internet-pornography-by-the-numbers.

8. The Box

1. Sonja Sharp, "'Scarlet Letter Statute': L.A.'s Adult Performers Strike Back against State Registry Bill," Los Angeles Times (Los Angeles Times, February 29, 2020), https://www.latimes.com/california/story/2020-02-29/porn-actors-los-angeles-state-registry-bill.

2. Ibid.

3. "Dirty Money: These Big Companies Use Porn Sites to Advertise Their Products," Fight the New Drug, May 1, 2018, https://fightthenewdrug.org/companies-that-use-porn-sites-to-advertise/.

4. "Joe Camel Advertising Campaign Violates Federal Law, FTC Says," Federal Trade Commission, May 28, 1997, https://www.ftc.gov/news-events/press-releases/1997/05/joe-camel-advertising-campaign-violates-federal-law-ftc-says.

9. Meet Ms. MEAT

1. Martin Amis, "Martin Amis on the Pornography Industry," The Guardian (Guardian News and Media, March 17, 2001), https://www.theguardian.com/books/2001/mar/17/society.martinamis1.

2. "Vanessa Williams Becomes First Black Miss America," History.com (A&E Television Networks, November 13, 2009), https://www.history.com/this-day-in-history/vanessa-williams-becomes-first-black-miss-america.

3. Jennifer Latson, "Why Vanessa Williams Gave Up Her Miss America Crown," Time (Time, July 23, 2015), https://time.com/3961120/miss-america-scandal-vanessa-williams/.

4. Ibid.

5. "Lisa Sparks Had Sex with 919 Men in a Day," Unreal Facts for Amazing facts, April 18, 2020, https://unrealfacts.com/a-woman-had-sex-with-919-men-in-a-day/.

6. Ibid.

7. "Wooden Horse (Device)," Wikipedia (Wikimedia Foundation, May 15, 2021), https://en.wikipedia.org/wiki/Wooden_horse_(device).

8. Ibid.

10. You are not in Control

1. Shoshana Zuboff, *The Age of Surveillance Capitalism: the Fight for the Future at the New Frontier of Power* (London: Profile Books, 2019).
2. Zuboff, 19.
3. *The Social Dilemma*.
4. "What Is the 'Invisible Hand' in Capitalism?" Investopedia (Investopedia, August 28, 2020), https://www.investopedia.com/ask/answers/012815/how-does-invisible-hand-affect-capitalist-economy.asp.
5. Patrick Keilty, "Desire by Design: Pornography as Technology Industry," *Porn Studies* 5, no. 3 (March 2018): pp. 338-342, https://doi.org/10.1080/23268743.2018.1483208.
6. Zuboff
7. Jaron Lanier, *Ten Arguments for Deleting Your Social Media Accounts Right Now* (New York, New York: Picador, Henry Holt and Company, 2019).
8. Chavie Lieber, "Tech Companies Use 'Persuasive Design' to Get Us Hooked. Psychologists Say It's Unethical.," Vox (Vox, August 8, 2018), https://www.vox.com/2018/8/8/17664580/persuasive-technology-psychology.
9. John Geirland, "Go with The Flow," Wired (Conde Nast, June 4, 2017), https://www.wired.com/1996/09/czik.
10. Ibid.
11. Alexis C. Madrigal, "The Machine Zone: This Is Where You Go When You Just Can't Stop Looking at Pictures on Facebook," The Atlantic (Atlantic Media Company, July 31, 2013), https://www.theatlantic.com/technology/archive/2013/07/the-machine-zone-this-is-where-you-go-when-you-just-cant-stop-looking-at-pictures-on-facebook/278185/.
12. Ibid.
13. Ibid.
14. Ibid.
15. Ibid.
16. *The Social Dilemma*, Netflix, 2020, https://www.netflix.com/title/81254224.
17. Ibid.
18. Ibid.
19. John Cheney-Lippold, "A New Algorithmic Identity," *Theory, Culture & Society* 28, no. 6 (2011): pp. 164-181, https://doi.org/10.1177/0263276411424420.
20. *The Matrix* (Warner Brothers, 1999).
21. Keilty, "Desire by Design."

11. The Bait

1. Zuboff, 28-30.
2. Ibid, 67-68.
3. Ibid, 76-78.
4. Ibid.

5. Ibid.
6. The Social Dilemma.

12. The Trigger

1.· Aaron O'Neill, "United States: Child Mortality Rate 1800-2020," Statista, March 19, 2021, https://www.statista.com/statistics/1041693/united-states-all-time-child-mortality-rate/.
2. "Study Finds Male and Female Brains Respond Differently to Visual Stimuli," ScienceDaily,   March   16,   2004,   http://www.sciencedaily.com/releas-es/2004/03/040316072953.htm.
3. Ibid.
4. Ibid.
5. "How Porn Can Change the Brain," Fight the New Drug, June 9, 2021, https://fightthenewdrug.org/how-porn-can-change-the-brain/.
6. Matt Morrissey, "How Early Porn Exposure Traumatizes Boys and Fuels an Unhealthy Perception of Masculinity," Fight the New Drug, May 5, 2021, https://fightthenewdrug.org/matt-morrissey-how-porn-exposure-traumatizes-boys/.
7. Alexandra Katehakis, "Effects of Porn on Adolescent Boys," Psychology Today (Sussex Publishers, July 28, 2011), https://www.psychologytoday.com/us/blog/sex-lies-trauma/201107/effects-porn-adolescent-boys.

13. The Door

1. Morten L Kringelbach and Kent C Berridge, "The Neuroscience of Happiness and Pleasure," *Social Research* 77, no. 2 (2010): pp. 659-678.
2. Ibid.
3. "Why Consuming Porn Is an Escalating Behavior," Fight the New Drug, June 26, 2018,   https://fightthenewdrug.org/why-consuming-porn-is-an-escalating-behavior/.
4. Ibid.
5. Ibid.
6. Ibid.
7. Ibid.
8. K. K. Pitchers et al., "DeltaFosB in the Nucleus Accumbens Is Critical for Reinforcing Effects of Sexual Reward," *Genes, Brain and Behavior* 9, no. 7 (July 2010): pp. 831-840, https://doi.org/10.1111/j.1601-183x.2010.00621.x.
9. E. J. Nestler, M. Barrot, and D. W. Self, "DeltaFosB: A Sustained Molecular Switch for Addiction," *Proceedings of the National Academy of Sciences* 98, no. 20 (2001): pp. 11042-11046, https://doi.org/10.1073/pnas.191352698.
10. Ibid.
11. ScienceDaily, "Male and Female Brains Respond Differently."

12. Jennifer P. Schneider, "Effects of Cybersex Addiction on the Family: Results of a Survey," *Sexual Addiction & Compulsivity* 7, no. 1-2 (2000): pp. 31-58, https://doi.org/10.1080/10720160008400206.

13. "How Porn Can Hurt a Consumer's Partner," Fight the New Drug, June 10, 2021, https://fightthenewdrug.org/how-porn-can-hurt-a-consumers-partner/#c4.

14. Morrissey, "Early Porn Exposure."

15. Rachel Ehmke, "How Using Social Media Affects Teenagers," Child Mind Institute, May 10, 2021, https://childmind.org/article/how-using-social-media-affects-teenagers/.

16. The Social Dilemma.

17. "One in 10 Visitors to Hardcore Porn Sites Is Under 10 Years Old, Study Shows," Fight the New Drug, July 30, 2018, https://fightthenewdrug.org/data-says-one-in-10-visitors-to-porn-sites-are-under-10-years-old/.

14. The Lock

1. Christian Keysers and Valeria Gazzola, "Hebbian Learning and Predictive Mirror Neurons for Actions, Sensations and Emotions," *Philosophical Transactions of the Royal Society B: Biological Sciences* 369, no. 1644 (May 2014): p. 20130175, https://doi.org/10.1098/rstb.2013.0175.

2. Kenji Katahira et al., "EEG Correlates of the Flow State: A Combination of Increased Frontal Theta and Moderate Frontocentral Alpha Rhythm in the Mental Arithmetic Task," *Frontiers in Psychology* 9 (September 2018), https://doi.org/10.3389/fpsyg.2018.00300.

3. F. Du et al., "Tightly Coupled Brain Activity and Cerebral ATP Metabolic Rate," *Proceedings of the National Academy of Sciences* 105, no. 17 (2008): pp. 6409-6414, https://doi.org/10.1073/pnas.0710766105.

15. The Cage

1. Justin J Lehmiller, "Penile Dysmorphic Disorder: When Penis Size Concerns Get Out of Control," Sex and Psychology (Sex and Psychology, September 4, 2015), https://www.lehmiller.com/blog/2015/8/24/penile-dysmorphic-disorder-when-penis-size-concerns-get-out-of-control.

2. Colin Drury, "'I Wanted a Truncheon in My Pants': the Rise of the Penis Extension," The Guardian (Guardian News and Media, September 22, 2018), https://www.theguardian.com/lifeandstyle/2018/sep/22/penis-extension-wanted-truncheon-in-pants-rise.

3. Ibid.

4. Marleen J. Klaassen and Jochen Peter, "Gender (In)Equality in Internet Pornography: A Content Analysis of Popular Pornographic Internet Videos," *The Journal of Sex Research* 52, no. 7 (2014): pp. 721-735, https://doi.org/10.1080/00224499.2014.976781.

5. Vincent Estellon and Harold Mouras, "Sexual Addiction: Insights from Psycho-analysis and Functional Neuroimaging," *Socioaffective Neuroscience & Psychology* 2, no. 1 (2012): p. 11814, https://doi.org/10.3402/snp.v2i0.11814.
6. Valerie L. Kinner, Oliver T. Wolf, and Christian J. Merz, "Cortisol Increases the Return of Fear by Strengthening Amygdala Signaling in Men," *Psychoneuroendocrinology* 91 (2018): pp. 79-85, https://doi.org/10.1016/j.psyneuen.2018.02.020.
7. Brené Brown, "Shame v. Guilt," Brené Brown, August 21, 2019, https://brenebrown.com/blog/2013/01/14/shame-v-guilt.

16. The Chains That Bind

1. Brian Park et al., "Is Internet Pornography Causing Sexual Dysfunctions? A Review with Clinical Reports," *Behavioral Sciences* 6, no. 3 (May 2016): p. 17, https://doi.org/10.3390/bs6030017.
2. T. N. Vidya, "Supernormal Stimuli and Responses," *Resonance* 23, no. 8 (2018): pp. 853-860, https://doi.org/10.1007/s12045-018-0688-x.
3. Park "Sexual Dysfunctions?"
4. "How Porn Can Change the Brain," Fight the New Drug, June 9, 2021, https://fightthenewdrug.org/how-porn-can-change-the-brain/.
5. Mike J.F. Robinson and Kent C. Berridge, "Instant Transformation of Learned Repulsion into Motivational 'Wanting,'" *Current Biology* 23, no. 4 (2013): pp. 282-289, https://doi.org/10.1016/j.cub.2013.01.016.
6. Keilty, "Desire by Design."
7. Răzvan Mureşan, "One in 10 Visitors of Porn Sites Is under 10 Years Old," HOTforSecurity, September 29, 2016, https://hotforsecurity.bitdefender.com/blog/one-in-10-visitors-of-porn-sites-is-under-10-years-old-16675.html.
8. John Schwartz, "The Pornography Industry vs. Digital Pirates," The New York Times (The New York Times, February 8, 2004), https://www.nytimes.com/2004/02/08/business/the-pornography-industry-vs-digital-pirates.html.

17. The Box

1. "Ashley Madison Data Breach," Wikipedia (Wikimedia Foundation, February 16, 2021), https://en.wikipedia.org/wiki/Ashley_Madison_data_breach.
2. Ibid.
3. Charles J Orlando, "I Was Hacked on Ashley Madison – But It's You Who Should Be Ashamed," Yahoo! (Yahoo!, July 23, 2015), https://www.yahoo.com/lifestyle/i-was-hacked-on-ashley-madison-but-its-you-who-124846903673.html.
4. Laurie Segall, "Pastor Outed on Ashley Madison Commits Suicide," CNNMoney (Cable News Network, September 8, 2015), https://money.cnn.com/2015/09/08/technology/ashley-madison-suicide/index.html.
5. Ibid.
6. Brian Merchant, "Your Porn Is Watching You," Vice, April 6, 2015, https://www.vice.com/en/article/539485/your-porn-is-watching-you.

7. Mureşan, "One in 10."

8. Maria Teresa Valadas and Lucilia Eduarda Bravo, "De Clérambault's Syndrome Revisited: a Case Report of Erotomania in a Male," *BMC Psychiatry* 20, no. 1 (October 23, 2020), https://doi.org/10.1186/s12888-020-02921-5.

9. Ibid.

10. Ibid.

11. Lisa Damour, "We Know It Harms Kids to See Smoking on TV. What About Rape?" The New York Times (The New York Times, September 12, 2019), https://www.nytimes.com/2019/09/12/well/family/we-know-it-harms-kids-to-see-smoking-on-tv-what-about-rape.html.

12. Vanessa Romo, "Netflix Promises to Quit Smoking On (Most) Original Programming," NPR (NPR, July 4, 2019), https://www.npr.org/2019/07/04/738719658/netflix-promises-to-quit-smoking-on-most-original-programming.

13. Ibid.

14. Neil M Malamuth and James V.P Check, "The Effects of Mass Media Exposure on Acceptance of Violence against Women: A Field Experiment," *Journal of Research in Personality* 15, no. 4 (1981): pp. 436-446, https://doi.org/10.1016/0092-6566(81)90040-4.

15. Eleanor Halls, "Who Are the 'Incels'? The Involuntary Celibates Who Want Women Punished," British GQ (British GQ, July 2, 2019), https://www.gq-magazine.co.uk/article/incel-meaning-explained.

16. Alice Hines, "How Many Bones Would You Break to Get Laid?" The Cut (New York Magazine, May 28, 2019), https://www.thecut.com/2019/05/incel-plastic-surgery.html.

17. Ibid.

18. "Online Poll Results Provide New Insights into Incel Community," Anti-Defamation League, September 10, 2020, https://www.adl.org/blog/online-poll-results-provide-new-insights-into-incel-community.

19. Sian Tomkinson Media and, Katie Attwell, and Tauel Harper, "'Incel' Violence is a Form of Extremism. It's Time We Treated it as a Security Threat," The Conversation, February 4, 2021, https://theconversation.com/incel-violence-is-a-form-of-extremism-its-time-we-treated-it-as-a-security-threat-138536.

20. "The Manifesto of Elliot Rodger," The New York Times (The New York Times, May 25, 2014), https://www.nytimes.com/interactive/2014/05/25/us/shooting-document.html.

21. Ibid.

22. Ibid.

23. Ibid.

24. Tanya Basu, "The 'Manosphere' Is Getting More Toxic as Angry Men Join the Incels," MIT Technology Review (MIT Technology Review, April 2, 2020), https://www.technologyreview.com/2020/02/07/349052/the-manosphere-is-getting-more-toxic-as-angry-men-join-the-incels/.

25. Manoel Ribeiro et al., "(PDF) The Evolution of the Manosphere Across the Web," ResearchGate, January 2020, https://www.researchgate.net/publication/338737324_The_Evolution_of_the_Manosphere_Across_the_Web.

26. Tanya Basu, "The 'Manosphere'."

27. "Texas Domestic Terrorism Threat Assessment" (Texas Department of Public Safety, January 6, 2020), https://www.dps.texas.gov/sites/default/files/documents/director_staff/media_and_communications/2020/txterrorthreatassessment.pdf.

28. "Press Releases and Media Resources: Pornhub," Pornhub Porn Videos, 2020, https://www.pornhub.com/press.

18. No More Dead Meat

1. Nicholas Kristof, "The Children of Pornhub," The New York Times (The New York Times, December 4, 2020), https://www.nytimes.com/2020/12/04/opinion/sunday/pornhub-rape-trafficking.html.

19. Shutting Down the Trap

1. The Social Dilemma.

2. Richard L Merrill, "PDF" (Houston, Texas, April 20, 2009).

3. "How to Avoid Buying Blood Diamonds," Brilliance.com, June 5, 2018, https://www.brilliance.com/diamonds/avoid-buying-blood-diamonds.

4. Stern, "She was Fired."

5. Ibid.

6. Ibid.

7. "FAQs," Arkansas Department of Labor and Licensing, November 16, 2020, https://www.labor.arkansas.gov/resources/faqs/.

8. Stern, "She Was Fired From Taco Bell."

9. Kristof, "The Children of Pornhub."

WORKS CITED

"2018 Year in Review." Pornhub Insights. Pornhub, December 11, 2018. https://www.pornhub.com/insights/2018-year-in-review.

"The 2019 Year in Review." Pornhub Insights. Pornhub, December 11, 2019. https://www.pornhub.com/insights/2019-year-in-review.

"Advertising and Promotion." Center for Tobacco Products. U.S. Food and Drug Administration, n.d. https://www.fda.gov/tobacco-products/products-guidance-regulations/advertising-and-promotion.

Amis, Martin. "Martin Amis on the Pornography Industry." The Guardian. Guardian News and Media, March 17, 2001. https://www.theguardian.com/books/2001/mar/17/society.martinamis1.

"Ashley Madison Data Breach." Wikipedia. Wikimedia Foundation, February 16, 2021. https://en.wikipedia.org/wiki/Ashley_Madison_data_breach.

Ayala, Eva-Marie. "Dallas Teacher's Past as Porn Actress Led to Her Firing, She Says." Dallas News. The Dallas Morning News, August 25,

2019. https://www.dallasnews.com/news/education/2017/02/01/dallas-teacher-s-past-as-porn-actress-led-to-her-firing-she-says/.

Basu, Tanya. "The 'Manosphere' Is Getting More Toxic as Angry Men Join the Incels." MIT Technology Review. MIT Technology Review, April 2, 2020. https://www.technologyreview.com/2020/02/07/349052/the-manosphere-is-getting-more-toxic-as-angry-men-join-the-incels/.

Berridge, Kent C., and Terry E. Robinson. "Liking, Wanting, and the Incentive-Sensitization Theory of Addiction." *American Psychologist* 71, no. 8 (2016): 670–79. https://doi.org/10.1037/amp0000059.

Biron, Bethany. "Beauty Has Blown up to Be a $532 Billion Industry - and Analysts Say That These 4 Trends Will Make It Even Bigger." Business Insider. Business Insider, July 9, 2019. https://www.businessinsider.com/beauty-multibillion-industry-trends-future-2019-7.

Brown, Annie. "Scots Women Warned Sex Webcamming Is Not Easy Way to Make Money during Lockdown." Daily Record. The Daily Record and Sunday Mail, May 7, 2020. https://www.dailyrecord.co.uk/news/scottish-news/women-turning-sex-webcamming-make-21993210.

Brown, Brené. "Shame v. Guilt." Brené Brown, August 21, 2019. https://brenebrown.com/blog/2013/01/14/shame-v-guilt.

Cheney-Lippold, John. "A New Algorithmic Identity." *Theory, Culture & Society* 28, no. 6 (2011): 164–81. https://doi.org/10.1177/0263276411424420.

Damour, Lisa. "We Know It Harms Kids to See Smoking on TV. What About Rape?" The New York Times. The New York Times, September 12, 2019. https://www.nytimes.com/2019/09/12/well/family/we-know-it-harms-kids-to-see-smoking-on-tv-what-about-rape.html.

"Dirty Money: These Big Companies Use Porn Sites To Advertise Their Products." Fight the New Drug, May 1, 2018. https://fightthenewdrug.org/companies-that-use-porn-sites-to-advertise/.

"Disaster Loan Assistance." SBA, n.d. https://covid19relief.sba.gov/.

"Dissociative Disorders." NAMI, n.d. https://www.nami.org/About-Mental-Illness/Mental-Health-Conditions/Dissociative-Disorders.

Downs, Claire. "Why Is Everybody Suddenly Selling Their Nudes?" ELLE. ELLE Magazine, May 15, 2020. https://www.elle.com/culture/a32459935/onlyfans-sex-work-influencers/.

Drolet, Gabrielle, and Shane O'Neill. "The Year Sex Work Came Home." The New York Times. The New York Times, April 10, 2020. https://www.nytimes.com/2020/04/10/style/camsoda-onlyfans-streaming-sex-coronavirus.html.

Drury, Colin. "'I Wanted a Truncheon in My Pants': the Rise of the Penis Extension." The Guardian. Guardian News and Media, September 22, 2018. https://www.theguardian.com/lifeandstyle/2018/sep/22/penis-extension-wanted-truncheon-in-pants-rise.

Du, F., X.-H. Zhu, Y. Zhang, M. Friedman, N. Zhang, K. Ugurbil, and W. Chen. "Tightly Coupled Brain Activity and Cerebral ATP Metabolic Rate." *Proceedings of the National Academy of Sciences* 105, no. 17 (2008): 6409–14. https://doi.org/10.1073/pnas.0710766105.

Ehmke, Rachel. "How Using Social Media Affects Teenagers." Child Mind Institute, May 10, 2021. https://childmind.org/article/how-using-social-media-affects-teenagers/.

"Erotomania: Causes, Symptoms, Diagnosis, and Treatment." Medical News Today. MediLexicon International, 2017. https://www.medicalnewstoday.com/articles/319145.

Estellon, Vincent, and Harold Mouras. "Sexual Addiction: Insights from Psychoanalysis and Functional Neuroimaging." *Socioaffective Neuroscience & Psychology* 2, no. 1 (2012): 11814. https://doi.org/10.3402/snp.v2i0.11814.

"FAQs." Arkansas Department of Labor and Licensing, November 16, 2020. https://www.labor.arkansas.gov/resources/faqs/.

Geirland, John. "Go With The Flow." Wired. Conde Nast, June 4, 2017. https://www.wired.com/1996/09/czik.

Germain, Thomas. "How a Photo's Hidden 'Exif' Data Exposes Your Personal Information." Consumer Reports, December 6, 2019. https://www.consumerreports.org/privacy/what-can-you-tell-from-photo-exif-data/.

Goodwin, Jazmin. "Mastercard, Visa and Discover Cut Ties with Pornhub Following Allegations of Child Abuse." CNN. Cable News Network, December 14, 2020. https://www.cnn.com/2020/12/14/business/mastercard-visa-discover-pornhub/index.html.

Halls, Eleanor. "Who Are the 'Incels'? The Involuntary Celibates Who Want Women Punished." British GQ. British GQ, July 2, 2019. https://www.gq-magazine.co.uk/article/incel-meaning-explained.

Hines, Alice. "How Many Bones Would You Break to Get Laid?" The Cut. New York Magazine, May 28, 2019. https://www.thecut.com/2019/05/incel-plastic-surgery.html.

"History of the Surgeon General's Report on Smoking and Health." Centers for Disease Control and Prevention. Centers for Disease Control and Prevention, November 15, 2019. https://www.cdc.gov/tobacco/data_statistics/sgr/history/index.htm.

"How Porn Affects Sexual Tastes." Fight the New Drug, June 26, 2018. https://fightthenewdrug.org/how-porn-affects-sexual-tastes/.

"How Porn Can Change the Brain." Fight the New Drug, June 9, 2021. https://fightthenewdrug.org/how-porn-can-change-the-brain/.

"How Porn Can Hurt a Consumer's Partner." Fight the New Drug, June 10, 2021. https://fightthenewdrug.org/how-porn-can-hurt-a-consumers-partner/#c4.

"How to Avoid Buying Blood Diamonds." Brilliance.com, June 5, 2018. https://www.brilliance.com/diamonds/avoid-buying-blood-diamonds.

"Human Trafficking." The United States Department of Justice, November 9, 2018. https://www.justice.gov/humantrafficking.

"Internet Pornography by the Numbers." Webroot. An Opentext Company, n.d. https://www.webroot.com/us/en/resources/tips-articles/internet-pornography-by-the-numbers.

Italiano, Laura. "Prostitute Finally Gets Justice in Rape." New York Post. New York Post, April 16, 2010. https://nypost.com/2010/04/16/prostitute-finally-gets-justice-in-rape/.

"Joe Camel Advertising Campaign Violates Federal Law, FTC Says." Federal Trade Commission, May 28, 1997. https://www.ftc.gov/news-events/press-releases/1997/05/joe-camel-advertising-campaign-violates-federal-law-ftc-says.

Katahira, Kenji, Yoichi Yamazaki, Chiaki Yamaoka, Hiroaki Ozaki, Sayaka Nakagawa, and Noriko Nagata. "EEG Correlates of the Flow State: A Combination of Increased Frontal Theta and Moderate Frontocentral Alpha Rhythm in the Mental Arithmetic Task." *Frontiers in Psychology* 9 (2018). https://doi.org/10.3389/fpsyg.2018.00300.

Katehakis, Alexandra. "Effects of Porn on Adolescent Boys." Psychology Today. Sussex Publishers, July 28, 2011. https://www.psychologytoday.com/us/blog/sex-lies-trauma/201107/effects-porn-adolescent-boys.

Keilty, Patrick. "Desire by Design: Pornography as Technology Industry." *Porn Studies* 5, no. 3 (2018): 338–42. https://doi.org/10.1080/23268743.2018.1483208.

Keysers, Christian, and Valeria Gazzola. "Hebbian Learning and Predictive Mirror Neurons for Actions, Sensations and Emotions." *Philosophical Transactions of the Royal Society B: Biological Sciences* 369, no. 1644 (2014): 20130175. https://doi.org/10.1098/rstb.2013.0175.

Kinner, Valerie L., Oliver T. Wolf, and Christian J. Merz. "Cortisol Increases the Return of Fear by Strengthening Amygdala Signaling in Men." *Psychoneuroendocrinology* 91 (2018): 79–85. https://doi.org/10.1016/j.psyneuen.2018.02.020.

Klaassen, Marleen J., and Joaq chen Peter. "Gender (In)Equality in Internet Pornography: A Content Analysis of Popular Pornographic Internet Videos." *The Journal of Sex Research* 52, no. 7 (2014): 721–35. https://doi.org/10.1080/00224499.2014.976781.

Kringelbach, Morten L, and Kent C Berridge. "The Neuroscience of Happiness and Pleasure." *Social Research* 77, no. 2 (2010): 659–78. PMID: 22068342; PMCID: PMC3008658.

Kristof, Nicholas. "The Children of Pornhub." The New York Times. The New York Times, December 4, 2020. https://www.nytimes.com/2020/12/04/opinion/sunday/pornhub-rape-trafficking.html.

Lanier, Jaron. *Ten Arguments for Deleting Your Social Media Accounts Right Now*. New York, New York: Picador, Henry Holt and Company, 2019.

"The Latest on Our Commitment to Trust and Safety." Pornhub Porn Videos, n.d. https://www.pornhub.com/blog/11422.

Latson, Jennifer. "Why Vanessa Williams Gave Up Her Miss America Crown." Time. Time, July 23, 2015. https://time.com/3961120/miss-america-scandal-vanessa-williams/.

Lehmiller, Justin J. "Penile Dysmorphic Disorder: When Penis Size Concerns Get Out Of Control." Sex And Psychology. Sex And Psychology, September 4, 2015. https://www.lehmiller.com/blog/2015/8/24/penile-dysmorphic-disorder-when-penis-size-concerns-get-out-of-control.

Lieber, Chavie. "Tech Companies Use 'Persuasive Design' to Get Us Hooked. Psychologists Say It's Unethical." Vox. Vox, August 8, 2018. https://www.vox.com/2018/8/8/17664580/persuasive-technology-psychology.

"Lisa Sparks Had Sex with 919 Men in a Day." Unreal Facts for Amazing facts, April 18, 2020. https://unrealfacts.com/a-woman-had-sex-with-919-men-in-a-day/.

Little, Becky. "When Cigarette Companies Used Doctors to Push Smoking." History.com. A&E Television Networks, September 13, 2018. https://www.history.com/news/cigarette-ads-doctors-smoking-endorsement.

"Long Island Serial Killer." Wikipedia. Wikimedia Foundation, May 20, 2021. https://en.wikipedia.org/wiki/Long_Island_serial_killer.

Madrigal, Alexis C. "The Machine Zone: This Is Where You Go When You Just Can't Stop Looking at Pictures on Facebook." The Atlantic. Atlantic Media Company, July 31, 2013. https://www.theatlantic.com/technology/archive/2013/07/the-machine-zone-this-is-where-you-go-when-you-just-cant-stop-looking-at-pictures-on-facebook/278185/.

Malamuth, Neil M, and James V.P Check. "The Effects of Mass Media Exposure on Acceptance of Violence against Women: A Field Experiment." *Journal of Research in Personality* 15, no. 4 (1981): 436–46. https://doi.org/10.1016/0092-6566(81)90040-4.

"The Manifesto of Elliot Rodger." The New York Times. The New York Times, May 25, 2014. https://www.nytimes.com/interactive/2014/05/25/us/shooting-document.html.

Masnick, Mike. "Police Realizing That SESTA/FOSTA Made Their Jobs Harder; Sex Traffickers Realizing It's Made Their Job Easier." Techdirt, May 14, 2018. https://www.techdirt.com/articles/20180509/13450339810/police-realizing-that-sesta-fosta-made-their-jobs-harder-sex-traffickers-realizing-made-their-job-easier.shtml.

Merchant, Brian. "Your Porn Is Watching You." Vice, April 6, 2015. https://www.vice.com/en/article/539485/your-porn-is-watching-you.

Merrill, Richard L. "Ownership of Mineral Rights Under Texas Law." Houston, Texas: Fabio & Merrill, Attorneys at Law, April 20, 2009. https://www.fabiomerrill.com/wp-content/uploads/sites/374/2019/10/Ownership-of-Mineral-Rights-Under-Texas-Law.pdf

Montgomery, Blake. "OnlyFans Reporting 3.5 Million New Signups in March, 60,000 of Them New Creators, per an Email from the Company. In the First Two Weeks of March Alone That Was a 75% Increase from the Normal Level." Twitter. Twitter, March 31, 2020. https://twitter.com/blakersdozen/status/1245072167689060353?lang=en.

Morrissey, Matt. "How Early Porn Exposure Traumatizes Boys and Fuels an Unhealthy Perception of Masculinity." Fight the New Drug,

May 5, 2021. https://fightthenewdrug.org/matt-morrissey-how-porn-exposure-traumatizes-boys/.

MUREȘAN, Răzvan. "One in 10 Visitors of Porn Sites Is under 10 Years Old." HOTforSecurity, September 29, 2016. https://hotforsecurity.bitdefender.com/blog/one-in-10-visitors-of-porn-sites-is-under-10-years-old-16675.html.

Nestler, E. J., M. Barrot, and D. W. Self. "DeltaFosB: A Sustained Molecular Switch for Addiction." *Proceedings of the National Academy of Sciences* 98, no. 20 (2001): 11042–46. https://doi.org/10.1073/pnas.191352698.

Oh-Willeke, Andrew. "Court: Firing Woman Due To Prior Porn Shoot Legal." The Colorado Independent, May 17, 2007. https://www.coloradoindependent.com/2007/05/17/court-firing-woman-due-to-prior-porn-shoot-legal/.

"One in 10 Visitors to Hardcore Porn Sites Is Under 10 Years Old, Study Shows." Fight the New Drug, July 30, 2018. https://fightthenewdrug.org/data-says-one-in-10-visitors-to-porn-sites-are-under-10-years-old/.

O'Neill, Aaron. "United States: Child Mortality Rate 1800-2020." Statista, March 19, 2021. https://www.statista.com/statistics/1041693/united-states-all-time-child-mortality-rate/.

"Online Poll Results Provide New Insights into Incel Community." Anti-Defamation League, September 10, 2020. https://www.adl.org/blog/online-poll-results-provide-new-insights-into-incel-community.

Orlando, Charles J. "I Was Hacked On Ashley Madison - But It's You Who Should Be Ashamed." Yahoo! Yahoo!, July 23, 2015. https://www.yahoo.com/lifestyle/i-was-hacked-on-ashley-madison-but-its-you-who-124846903673.html.

Palmer, Ewan, Billy Binion, and James R. Copland. "Sex Workers Say the Online Market Is Saturated with Performers and Fans Are Canceling Subscriptions during Coronavirus Pandemic." Newsweek, April 17, 2020. https://www.newsweek.com/coronavirus-sex-workers-cam-girls-online-1498024.

Park, Brian, Gary Wilson, Jonathan Berger, Matthew Christman, Bryn Reina, Frank Bishop, Warren Klam, and Andrew Doan. "Is Internet Pornography Causing Sexual Dysfunctions? A Review with Clinical Reports." *Behavioral Sciences* 6, no. 3 (2016): 17. https://doi.org/10.3390/bs6030017.

Perrin, Ben. "Hope Barden: Sex Role-Play Death Prompts Law Change Plea." BBC News. BBC, July 6, 2019. https://www.bbc.com/news/uk-england-stoke-staffordshire-48790961.

Pitchers, K. K., K. S. Frohmader, V. Vialou, E. Mouzon, E. J. Nestler, M. N. Lehman, and L. M. Coolen. "DeltaFosB in the Nucleus Accumbens Is Critical for Reinforcing Effects of Sexual Reward." *Genes, Brain and Behavior* 9, no. 7 (2010): 831–40. https://doi.org/10.1111/j.1601-183x.2010.00621.x.

"Pornhub Sets Standard for Safety and Security Policies Across Tech and Social Media; Announces Industry-Leading Measures for Verification, Moderation and Detection." Pornhub Porn Videos. Pornhub, February 2, 2021. https://www.pornhub.com/press/show?id=2172.

"Pornography Addiction." Sergen's Medical Dictionary. Farlex, 2012. https://medical-dictionary.thefreedictionary.com/Pornography+addiction.

"Press Releases and Media Resources: Pornhub." Pornhub Porn Videos, 2020. https://www.pornhub.com/press.

Ribeiro, Manoel, Savvas Zannettou, Stephanie Greenberg, Summer

Long, Gianluca Stringhini, Emiliano De Cristofaro, Barry Bradlyn, and Jeremy Blackburn. "(PDF) The Evolution of the Manosphere Across the Web." ResearchGate, January 2020. https://www. researchgate.net/publication/ 338737324_The_Evolution_of_the_Manosphere_Across_the_Web. To appear at the 15th International AAAI Conference on Web and Social Media (ICWSM 2021).

Robinson, Mike J.F., and Kent C. Berridge. "Instant Transformation of Learned Repulsion into Motivational 'Wanting.'" *Current Biology* 23, no. 4 (2013): 282–89. https://doi.org/10.1016/j.cub.2013.01.016.

Romo, Vanessa. "Netflix Promises To Quit Smoking On (Most) Original Programming." NPR. NPR, July 4, 2019. https://www.npr.org/2019/ 07/04/738719658/netflix-promises-to-quit-smoking-on-most-original-programming.

Schneider, Jennifer P. "Effects of Cybersex Addiction on the Family: Results of a Survey." *Sexual Addiction & Compulsivity* 7, no. 1-2 (2000): 31–58. https://doi.org/10.1080/10720160008400206.

Schwartz, John. "The Pornography Industry vs. Digital Pirates." The New York Times. The New York Times, February 8, 2004. https:// www.nytimes.com/2004/02/08/business/the-pornography-industry-vs-digital-pirates.html.

Segall, Laurie. "Pastor Outed on Ashley Madison Commits Suicide." CNNMoney. Cable News Network, September 8, 2015. https://money. cnn.com/2015/09/08/technology/ashley-madison-suicide/index.html.

Sharp, Sonja. "'Scarlet Letter Statute': L.A.'s Adult Performers Strike Back against State Registry Bill." Los Angeles Times. Los Angeles Times, February 29, 2020. https://www.latimes.com/california/story/ 2020-02-29/porn-actors-los-angeles-state-registry-bill.

The Social Dilemma. Netflix, 2020. https://www.netflix.com/ title/81254224.

Steadman, Otillia. "Her Colleagues Watched Her OnlyFans Account At Work. When Bosses Found Out, They Fired Her." BuzzFeed News. BuzzFeed News, September 29, 2020. https://www.buzzfeednews.com/ article/otilliasteadman/mechanic-fired-onlyfans-account-indiana.

Stern, Marlow. "She Was Fired From Taco Bell for Being in Porn." The Daily Beast. The Daily Beast Company, January 19, 2021. https:// www.thedailybeast.com/lonna-wells-was-fired-from-taco-bell-for-being-in-porn.

"Study Finds Male And Female Brains Respond Differently To Visual Stimuli." ScienceDaily, March 16, 2004. http://www.sciencedaily.com/ releases/2004/03/040316072953.htm.

"Texas Domestic Terrorism Threat Assessment." Texas Department of Public Safety, January 6, 2020. https://www.dps.texas.gov/sites/ default/files/documents/director_staff/media_and_communications/ 2020/txterrorthreatassessment.pdf.

Tomkinson, Sian, Katie Atwell, and Tauel Harper. "'Incel' Violence Is a Form of Extremism. It's Time We Treated It as a Security Threat." The Conversation, February 4, 2021. https://theconversation.com/ incel-violence-is-a-form-of-extremism-its-time-we-treated-it-as-a-security-threat-138536.

Valadas, Maria Teresa, and Lucilia Eduarda Bravo. "De Clérambault's Syndrome Revisited: a Case Report of Erotomania in a Male." *BMC Psychiatry* 20, no. 1 (October 23, 2020). https://doi.org/10.1186/s12888-020-02921-5.

"Vanessa Williams Becomes First Black Miss America." History.com.

A&E Television Networks, November 13, 2009. https://www.history. com/this-day-in-history/vanessa-williams-becomes-first-black-miss-america.

Vidya, T. N. "Supernormal Stimuli and Responses." *Resonance* 23, no. 8 (2018): 853–60. https://doi.org/10.1007/s12045-018-0688-x.

Villa, Philip. *Roll, Red, Roll. Netflix*, 2018. https://www.netflix.com/ title/81087761.

Wachowski, Lilly, Lana Wachowski, and Joel Silver. *The Matrix*. Film. United States: Warner Brothers, 1999.

"What Is the 'Invisible Hand' in Capitalism?" Investopedia. Investo-pedia, August 28, 2020. https://www.investopedia.com/ask/answers/ 012815/how-does-invisible-hand-affect-capitalist-economy.asp.

"What Is 'SESTA/FOSTA'?" Hacking//Hustling. Hacking//Hustling, November 22, 2020. https://hackinghustling.org/what-is-sesta-fosta/.

"Why Consuming Porn Is An Escalating Behavior." Fight the New Drug, June 26, 2018. https://fightthenewdrug.org/why-consuming-porn-is-an-escalating-behavior/.

Wolfson, Sam. "Snapchat Photo Filters Linked to Rise in Cosmetic Surgery Requests." The Guardian. Guardian News and Media, August 9, 2018. https://www.theguardian.com/technology/2018/aug/ 08/snapchat-surgery-doctors-report-rise-in-patient-requests-to-look-filtered.

"Wooden Horse (Device)." Wikipedia. Wikimedia Foundation, May 15, 2021. https://en.wikipedia.org/wiki/Wooden_horse_(device).

"Xanax Addiction and Abuse - Addiction to Alprazolam." Addiction

Center. Addiction Center, March 25, 2021. https://www.addictioncenter.com/benzodiazepines/xanax/.

Zetter, Kim. "Hackers Finally Post Stolen Ashley Madison Data." Wired. Conde Nast, August 2015. https://www.wired.com/2015/08/happened-hackers-posted-stolen-ashley-madison-data.

Zillmann, Dolf, and Jennings Bryant. "Pornography's Impact on Sexual Satisfaction1." *Journal of Applied Social Psychology* 18, no. 5 (1988): 438–53. https://doi.org/10.1111/j.1559-1816.1988.tb00027.x.

Zuboff, Shoshana. *The Age of Surveillance Capitalism: the Fight for the Future at the New Frontier of Power*. London: Profile Books, 2019.

Printed in the USA
CPSIA information can be obtained
at www.ICGtesting.com
LVHW010737050923
757241LV00009B/246